Virtual Clinical Excursions—Psychiatric

prepared by

Ruth N. Grendell, DNSc, RN
Professor Emerita
Point Loma Nazarene University
San Diego, CA

Faculty
University of Phoenix

Curriculum Consultant

software developed by

Wolfsong Informatics, LLC
Tucson, Arizona

ELSEVIER

ELSEVIER

3251 Riverport Lane
Maryland Heights, Missouri 63043

VIRTUAL CLINICAL EXCURSIONS—PSYCHIATRIC

ISBN: 978-0-323-42966-5

Notice

Knowledge and best practice in this field are constantly changing. As new research and experience broaden our understanding, changes in research methods, professional practices, or medical treatment may become necessary.

Practitioners and researchers must always rely on their own experience and knowledge in evaluating and using any information, methods, compounds, or experiments described herein. In using such information or methods they should be mindful of their own safety and the safety of others, including parties for whom they have a professional responsibility.

With respect to any drug or pharmaceutical products identified, readers are advised to check the most current information provided (i) on procedures featured or (ii) by the manufacturer of each product to be administered, to verify the recommended dose or formula, the method and duration of administration, and contraindications. It is the responsibility of practitioners, relying on their own experience and knowledge of their patients, to make diagnoses, to determine dosages and the best treatment for each individual patient, and to take all appropriate safety precautions.

To the fullest extent of the law, neither the Publisher nor the authors, contributors, or editors, assume any liability for any injury and/or damage to persons or property as a matter of products liability, negligence or otherwise, or from any use or operation of any methods, products, instructions, or ideas contained in the material herein.

ISBN: 978-0-323-42966-5

Printed in the United States of America

Last digit is the print number: 9 8 7 6 5 4 3 2 1

Textbooks

Halter: Varcarolis' Foundations of Psychiatric Mental Health Nursing, 7th edition

Keltner: Psychiatric Nursing, 7th edition

Varcarolis: Essentials of Psychiatric Mental Health Nursing, 2nd edition Revised Reprint

Contents

Getting Set Up with VCE Online 1

A Quick Tour 3

A Detailed Tour 19

Reducing Medication Errors 31

Lesson 1   Mental Health and Mental Illness 37

Lesson 2   Cultural Competence Related to Mental Health Nursing 45

Lesson 3   The Nurse-Patient Relationship 53

Lesson 4   Stress 61

Lesson 5   Anxiety Disorders 69

Lesson 6   Depressive Disorders 77

Lesson 7   Personality Disorders 85

Lesson 8   Schizophrenia Spectrum and Other Psychotic Disorders 91

Lesson 9   Substance Related Disorders 103

Lesson 10   Eating Disorders 115

Lesson 11   Childhood and Neurodevelopmental Disorders 125

Lesson 12   Psychological Needs of the Older Adult 135

Lesson 13   Cognitive Disorders 147

Lesson 14   Sexual Disorders, Assault, and Violence 161

Lesson 15   Crisis and Disaster 175

GETTING SET UP WITH VCE ONLINE ————————————————

The product you have purchased is part of the Evolve Learning System. Please read the following information thoroughly to get started.

■ HOW TO ACCESS YOUR VCE RESOURCES ON EVOLVE

There are two ways to access your VCE Resources on Evolve:

1. If your instructor has enrolled you in your VCE Evolve Resources, you will receive an email with your registration details.

2. If your instructor has asked you to self-enroll in your VCE Evolve Resources, he or she will provide you with your Course ID (for example, 1479_jdoe73_0001). You will then need to follow the instructions at https://evolve.elsevier.com/cs/studentEnroll.html.

■ HOW TO ACCESS THE ONLINE VIRTUAL HOSPITAL

The online virtual hospital is available through the Evolve VCE Resources. There is no software to download or install: the online virtual hospital runs within your Internet browser, using a pop-up window.

■ TECHNICAL REQUIREMENTS

- Broadband connection (DSL or cable)
- 1024 x 768 screen resolution
- Mozilla Firefox 18.0, Internet Explorer 9.0, Google Chrome, or Safari 5 (or higher)
  Note: Pop-up blocking software/settings must be disabled.
- Adobe Acrobat Reader
- Additional technical requirements available at http://evolvesupport.elsevier.com

■ HOW TO ACCESS THE WORKBOOK

There are two ways to access the workbook portion of *Virtual Clinical Excursions:*

1. Print workbook
2. An electronic version of the workbook, available within the VCE Evolve Resources

■ TECHNICAL SUPPORT

Technical support for *Virtual Clinical Excursions* is available by visiting the Technical Support Center at http://evolvesupport.elsevier.com or by calling 1-800-222-9570 inside the United States and Canada.

Trademarks: Windows® and Macintosh® are registered trademarks.

A QUICK TOUR

Welcome to *Virtual Clinical Excursions—Psychiatric*, a virtual hospital setting in which you can work with multiple complex patient simulations and also learn to access and evaluate the information resources that are essential for high-quality patient care. The virtual hospital, Pacific View Regional Hospital, has realistic architecture and access to patient rooms, a Nurses' Station, and a Medication Room.

■ BEFORE YOU START

Make sure you have your textbook nearby when you use *Virtual Clinical Excursions*. You will want to consult topic areas in your textbook frequently while working with the virtual hospital and workbook.

■ HOW TO SIGN IN

- Enter your name on the Student Nurse identification badge.
- Next, click the down arrow next to **Select Floor**. This drop-down menu lists only the floors on which there are currently patients with psychiatric nursing needs: Medical-Surgical, Obstetrics, Pediatrics, and Skilled Nursing. (For this quick tour, choose **Obstetrics**.)
- Now choose one of the four periods of care in which to work. In Periods of Care 1 through 3, you can actively engage in patient assessment, entry of data in the electronic patient record (EPR), and medication administration. Period of Care 4 presents the day in review. Highlight and click the appropriate period of care. (For this quick tour, choose **Period of Care 1**.)
- Click **Go**. This takes you to the Patient List screen (see the *How to Select a Patient* section below). Note that the virtual time is provided in the box at the lower left corner of the screen (0730, because we chose Period of Care 1).

Note: If you choose to work during Period of Care 4: 1900-2000, the Patient List screen is skipped because you are not able to visit patients or administer medications during the shift. Instead, you are taken directly to the Nurses' Station, where the records of all the patients on the floor are available for your review.

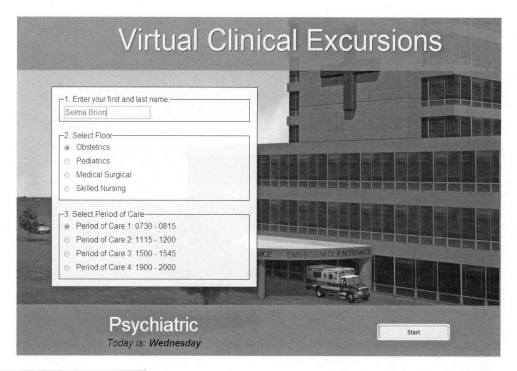

■ PATIENT LIST

OBSTETRICS UNIT

Dorothy Grant (Room 201)
30-week intrauterine pregnancy—A 25-year-old multipara Caucasian female admitted with abdominal trauma following a domestic violence incident. Her complications include preterm labor and extensive social issues such as acquiring safe housing for her family upon discharge.

Kelly Brady (Room 203)
26-week intrauterine pregnancy—A 35-year-old primigravida Caucasian female urgently admitted for progressive symptoms of preeclampsia. A history of inadequate coping with major life stressors leave her at risk for a recurrence of depression as she faces a diagnosis of HELLP syndrome and the delivery of a severely premature infant.

Laura Wilson (Room 206)
37-week intrauterine pregnancy—An 18-year-old primigravida Caucasian female urgently admitted after being found unconscious. Her complications include HIV-positive status and chronic polysubstance abuse. Unrealistic expectations of parenthood and living with a chronic illness, combined with strained family relations, prompt comprehensive social and psychiatric evaluations initiated on the day of simulation.

PEDIATRIC UNIT

Tiffany Sheldon (Room 305)
Anorexia nervosa—A 14-year-old Caucasian female admitted for dehydration, electrolyte imbalance, and malnutrition following a syncope episode at home. This patient has a history of eating disorders that have required multiple hospital admissions and have strained family dynamics between mother and daughter.

MEDICAL-SURGICAL UNIT

Harry George (Room 401)
Osteomyelitis—A 54-year-old Caucasian male admitted from a homeless shelter with an infected leg. He has complications of type 2 diabetes mellitus, alcohol abuse, nicotine addiction, poor pain control, and complex psychosocial issues.

Jacquline Catanazaro (Room 402)
Asthma—A 45-year-old Caucasian female admitted with an acute asthma exacerbation and suspected pneumonia. She has complications of chronic schizophrenia, noncompliance with medication therapy, obesity, and herniated disk.

SKILLED NURSING UNIT

Kathryn Doyle (Room 503)
Rehabilitation post left hip replacement—A 79-year-old Caucasian female admitted following a complicated recovery from an ORIF. She is experiencing symptoms of malnutrition and depression due to unstable family dynamics, placing her at risk for elder abuse.

Carlos Reyes (Room 504)
Rehabilitation status post myocardial infarction—An 81-year-old Hispanic male admitted for evaluation of the need for long-term care following an acute care hospital stay. Recent cognitive changes and a diagnosis of anxiety disorder contribute to stressful family dynamics and caregiver strain.

■ HOW TO SELECT A PATIENT

- You can choose one or more patients to work with from the Patient List by checking the box to the left of the patient name(s). For this quick tour, select Dorothy Grant. (In order to receive a scorecard for a patient, the patient must be selected before proceeding to the Nurses' Station.)
- Click on **Get Report** to the right of the medical records number (MRN) to view a summary of the patient's care during the 12-hour period before your arrival on the unit.
- After reviewing the report, click on **Go to Nurses' Station** in the right lower corner to begin your care. (*Note:* If you have been assigned to care for multiple patients, you can click on **Return to Patient List** to select and review the report for each additional patient before going to the Nurses' Station.)

Note: Even though the Patient List is initially skipped when you sign in to work for Period of Care 4, you can still access this screen if you wish to review the shift report for any of the patients. To do so, simply click on **Patient List** near the top left corner of the Nurses' Station (or click on the clipboard to the left of the Kardex). Then click on **Get Report** for the patient(s) whose care you are reviewing. This may be done during any period of care.

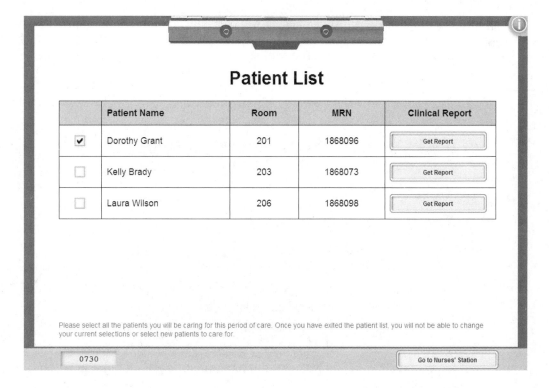

■ HOW TO FIND A PATIENT'S RECORDS

NURSES' STATION

Within the Nurses' Station, you will see:

1. A clipboard that contains the patient list for that floor.
2. A chart rack with patient charts labeled by room number, a notebook labeled Kardex, and a notebook labeled MAR (Medication Administration Record).
3. A desktop computer with access to the Electronic Patient Record (EPR).
4. A tool bar across the top of the screen that can also be used to access the Patient List, EPR, Chart, MAR, and Kardex. This tool bar is also accessible from each patient's room.
5. A Drug Guide containing information about the medications you are able to administer to your patients.
6. A Laboratory Guide containing normal value ranges for all laboratory tests you may come across in the virtual patient hospital.
7. A tool bar across the bottom of the screen that can be used to access the Floor Map, patient rooms, Medication Room, and Drug Guide.

As you run your cursor over an item, it will be highlighted. To select, simply click on the item. As you use these resources, you will always be able to return to the Nurses' Station by clicking on the **Return to Nurses' Station** bar located in the right lower corner of your screen.

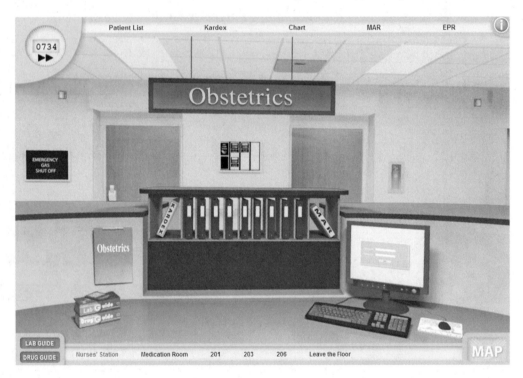

MEDICATION ADMINISTRATION RECORD (MAR)

The MAR icon located on the tool bar at the top of your screen accesses current 24-hour medications for each patient. Click on the icon and the MAR will open. (*Note:* You can also access the MAR by clicking on the MAR notebook on the far right side of the book rack in the center of the screen.) Within the MAR, tabs on the right side of the screen allow you to select patients by room number. Be careful to make sure you select the correct tab number for *your* patient rather than simply reading the first record that appears after the MAR opens. Each MAR sheet lists the following:

- Medications
- Route and dosage of each medication
- Times of administration of each medication

Note: The MAR changes each day. Expired MARs are stored in the patients' charts.

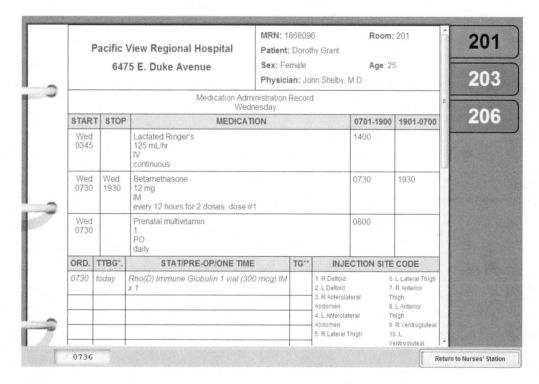

CHARTS

To access patient charts, either click on the **Chart** icon at the top of your screen or anywhere within the chart rack in the center of the Nurses' Station screen. When the close-up view appears, the individual charts are labeled by room number. To open a chart, click on the room number of the patient whose chart you wish to review. The patient's name and allergies will appear on the left side of the screen, along with a list of tabs on the right side of the screen, allowing you to view the following data:

- Allergies
- Physician's Orders
- Physician's Notes
- Nurse's Notes
- Laboratory Reports
- Diagnostic Reports
- Surgical Reports
- Consultations

- Patient Education
- History and Physical
- Nursing Admission
- Expired MARs
- Consents
- Mental Health
- Admissions
- Emergency Department

Information appears in real time. The entries are in reverse chronologic order, so use the down arrow at the right side of each chart page to scroll down to view previous entries. Flip from tab to tab to view multiple data fields or click on **Return to Nurses' Station** in the lower right corner of the screen to exit the chart.

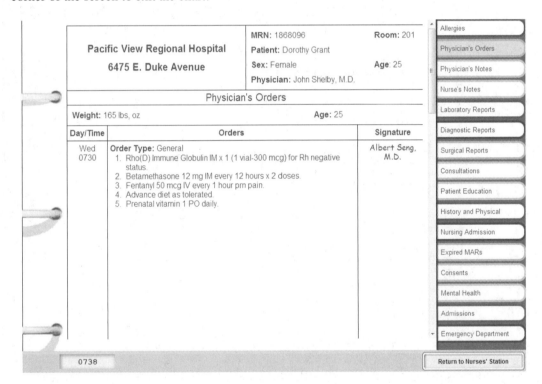

ELECTRONIC PATIENT RECORD (EPR)

The EPR can be accessed from the computer in the Nurses' Station or from the EPR icon located in the tool bar at the top of your screen. To access a patient's EPR:

- Click on either the computer screen or the **EPR** icon.
- Your username and password are automatically filled in.
- Click on **Login** to enter the EPR.
- *Note:* Like the MAR, the EPR is arranged numerically. Thus when you enter, you are initially shown the records of the patient in the lowest room number on the floor. To view the correct data for *your* patient, remember to select the correct room number, using the drop-down menu for the Patient field at the top left corner of the screen.

The EPR used in Pacific View Regional Hospital represents a composite of commercial versions being used in hospitals. You can access the EPR:

- to review existing data for a patient (by room number).
- to enter data you collect while working with a patient.

The EPR is updated daily, so no matter what day or part of a shift you are working, there will be a current EPR with the patient's data from the past days of the current hospital stay. This type of simulated EPR allows you to examine how data for different attributes have changed over time, as well as to examine data for all of a patient's attributes at a particular time. The EPR is fully functional (as it is in a real-life hospital). You can enter such data as blood pressure, breath sounds, and certain treatments. The EPR will not, however, allow you to enter data for a previous time period. Use the arrows at the bottom of the screen to move forward and backward in time.

Patient: 201		Category: Vital Signs			0733	
Name: Dorothy Grant	Wed 0345	Wed 0400	Wed 0500		Code Meanings	
PAIN: LOCATION	A	A	A	A	Abdomen	
PAIN: RATING	1	1	2-3	Ar	Arm	
PAIN: CHARACTERISTICS	A	D	I	B	Back	
PAIN: VOCAL CUES		NN	NN	C	Chest	
PAIN: FACIAL CUES			FC2	Ft	Foot	
PAIN: BODILY CUES				H	Head	
PAIN: SYSTEM CUES	NN			Hd	Hand	
PAIN: FUNCTIONAL EFFECTS				L	Left	
PAIN: PREDISPOSING FACTORS		NN	NN	Lg	Leg	
PAIN: RELIEVING FACTORS		NN	NN	Lw	Lower	
PCA				N	Neck	
TEMPERATURE (F)		97.6		NN	See Nurses notes	
TEMPERATURE (C)				OS	Operative site	
MODE OF MEASUREMENT		O		Or	See Physicians orders	
SYSTOLIC PRESSURE		126		PN	See Progress notes	
DIASTOLIC PRESSURE		66		R	Right	
BP MODE OF MEASUREMENT		NIBP		Up	Upper	
HEART RATE		72				
RESPIRATORY RATE		18				
SpO2 (%)						
BLOOD GLUCOSE						
WEIGHT						
HEIGHT						

Return to Nurses' Station

At the top of the EPR screen, you can choose patients by their room numbers. In addition, you have access to 17 different categories of patient data. To change patients or data categories, click the down arrow to the right of the room number or category.

The categories of patient data in the EPR are as follows:

- Vital Signs
- Respiratory
- Cardiovascular
- Neurologic
- Gastrointestinal
- Excretory
- Musculoskeletal
- Integumentary
- Reproductive
- Psychosocial
- Wounds and Drains
- Activity
- Hygiene and Comfort
- Safety
- Nutrition
- IV
- Intake and Output

Remember, each hospital selects its own codes. The codes used in the EPR at Pacific View Regional Hospital may be different from ones you have seen in your clinical rotations. Take some time to acquaint yourself with the codes. Within the Vital Signs category, click on any item in the left column (e.g., Pain: Characteristics). In the far-right column, you will see a list of code meanings for the possible findings and/or descriptors for that assessment area.

You will use the codes to record the data you collect as you work with patients. Click on the box in the last time column to the right of any item and wait for the code meanings applicable to that entry to appear. Select the appropriate code to describe your assessment findings and type it in the box. (*Note:* If no cursor appears within the box, click on the box again until the blue shading disappears and the blinking cursor appears.) Once the data are typed in this box, they are entered into the patient's record for this period of care only.

To leave the EPR, click on **Exit EPR** in the bottom right corner of the screen.

■ VISITING A PATIENT

From the Nurses' Station, click on the room number of the patient you wish to visit (in the tool bar at the bottom of your screen). Once you are inside the room, you will see a still photo of your patient in the top left corner. To verify that this is the correct patient, click on the **Check Armband** icon to the right of the photo. The patient's identification data will appear. If you click on **Check Allergies** (the next icon to the right), a list of the patient's allergies (if any) will replace the photo.

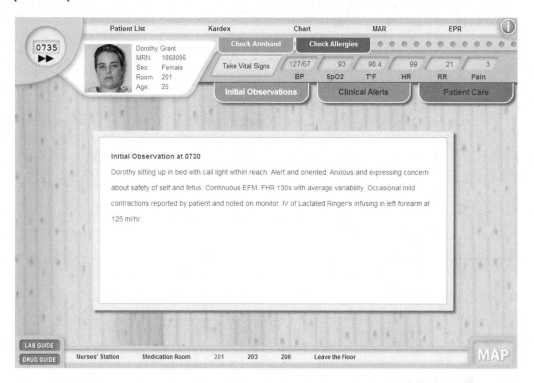

Also located in the patient's room are multiple icons you can use to assess the patient or the patient's medications. A virtual clock is provided in the upper left corner of the room to monitor your progress in real time. (*Note:* The fast-forward icon within the virtual clock will advance the time by 2-minute intervals when clicked.)

- The tool bar across the top of the screen allows you to check the **Patient List**, access the **EPR** to check or enter data, and view the patient's **Chart**, **MAR**, or **Kardex**.

- The **Take Vital Signs** icon allows you to measure the patient's up-to-the-minute blood pressure, oxygen saturation, temperature, heart rate, respiratory rate, and pain level.

- Each time you enter a patient's room, you are given an Initial Observation report to review (in the text box under the patient's photo). These notes are provided to give you a "look" at the patient as if you had just stepped into the room. You can also click on the **Initial Observations** icon to return to this box from other views within the patient's room. To the right of this icon is **Clinical Alerts**, a resource that allows you to make decisions about priority medication interventions based on emerging data collected in real time. Check this screen throughout your period of care to avoid missing critical information related to recently ordered or STAT medications.

- Clicking on **Patient Care** opens up three specific learning environments within the patient room: **Physical Assessment**, **Nurse-Client Interactions**, and **Medication Administration**.

- To perform a **Physical Assessment**, choose a body area (such as **Head & Neck**) from the column of yellow buttons. This activates a list of system subcategories for that body area (e.g., see **Sensory**, **Neurologic**, etc. in the green boxes). After you select the system you wish to evaluate, a brief description of the assessment findings will appear in a box to the right. A still photo provides a "snapshot" of how an assessment of this area might be done or what the finding might look like. For every body area, you can also click on **Equipment** on the right side of the screen.

• To the right of the Physical Assessment icon is **Nurse-Client Interactions**. Clicking on this icon will reveal the times and titles of any videos available for viewing. (*Note:* If the video you wish to see is not listed, this means you have not yet reached the correct virtual time to view that video. Check the virtual clock; you may return to access the video once its designated time has occurred—as long as you do so within the same period of care. Or you can click on the fast-forward icon within the virtual clock to advance the time by 2-minute intervals. You will then need to click again on **Patient Care** and **Nurse-Client Interactions** to refresh the screen.) To view a listed video, click on the white arrow to the right of the video title. Use the control buttons below the video to start, stop, pause, rewind, or fast-forward the action or to mute the sound.

• **Medication Administration** is the pathway that allows you to review and administer medications to a patient after you have prepared them in the Medication Room. This process is also addressed further in the *How to Prepare Medications* section below and in *Medications* in **A Detailed Tour**. For additional hands-on practice, see *Reducing Medication Errors* below **A Quick Tour** and **A Detailed Tour** in your resources.

■ HOW TO QUIT, CHANGE PATIENTS, CHANGE FLOORS, OR CHANGE PERIODS OF CARE

How to Quit: From most screens, you may click the **Leave the Floor** icon on the bottom tool bar to the right of the patient room numbers. (*Note:* From some screens, you will first need to click an **Exit** button or **Return to Nurses' Station** before clicking **Leave the Floor**.) When the Floor Menu appears, click **Exit** to leave the program.

How to Change Patients, Floors, or Periods of Care: To change patients, simply click on the new patient's room number. (You cannot receive a scorecard for a new patient, however, unless you have already selected that patient on the Patient List screen.) To change to a new period of care, to change floors, or to restart the virtual clock, click on **Leave the Floor** and then on **Restart the Program**.

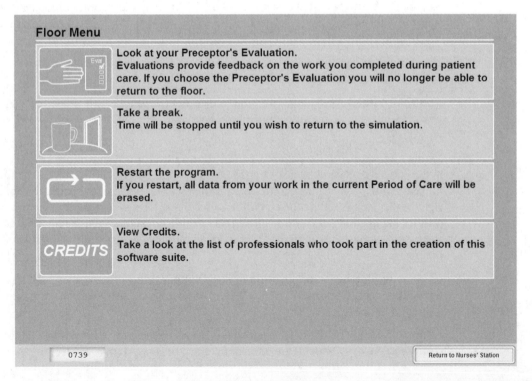

■ HOW TO PREPARE MEDICATIONS

From the Nurses' Station or the patient's room, you can access the Medication Room by clicking on the icon in the tool bar at the bottom of your screen to the left of the patient room numbers.

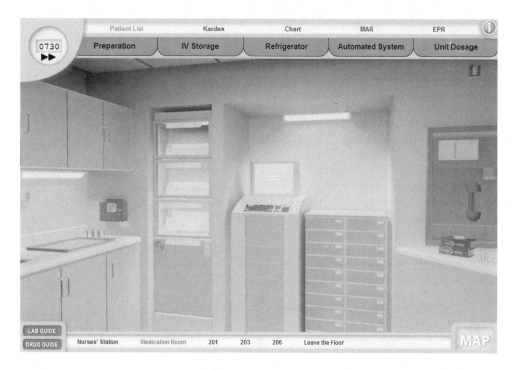

In the Medication Room you have access to the following (from left to right):

- A preparation area is located on the counter under the cabinets. To begin the medication preparation process, click on the tray on the counter or click on the **Preparation** icon at the top of the screen. The next screen leads you through a specific sequence (called the Preparation Wizard) to prepare medications one at a time for administration to a patient. However, no medication has been selected at this time. We will do this while working with a patient in **A Detailed Tour**. To exit this screen, click on **View Medication Room**.

- To the right of the cabinets (and above the refrigerator), IV storage bins are provided. Click on the bins themselves or on the **IV Storage** icon at the top of the screen. The bins are labeled **Microinfusion**, **Small Volume**, and **Large Volume**. Click on an individual bin to see a list of its contents. If you needed to prepare an IV medication at this time, you could click on the medication and its label would appear to the right under the patient's name. (*Note:* You can **Open** and **Close** any medication label by clicking the appropriate icon.) Next, you would click **Put Medication on Tray**. If you ever change your mind or decide that you have put the incorrect medication on the tray, you can reverse your actions by highlighting the medication on the tray and then clicking **Put Medication in Bin**. Click **Close Bin** in the right bottom corner to exit. **View Medication Room** brings you back to a full view of the entire room.

- A refrigerator is located under the IV storage bins to hold any medications that must be stored below room temperature. Click on the refrigerator door or on the **Refrigerator** icon at the top of the screen. Then click on the close-up view of the door to access the medications. When you are finished, click **Close Door** and then **View Medication Room**.

- To prepare controlled substances, click the **Automated System** icon at the top of the screen or click the computer monitor located to the right of the IV storage bins. A login screen will appear; your name and password are automatically filled in. Click **Login**. Select the patient for whom you wish to access medications; then select the correct medication drawer to open (they are stored alphabetically). Click **Open Drawer**, highlight the proper medication, and choose **Put Medication on Tray**. When you are finished, click **Close Drawer** and then **View Medication Room**.

- Next to the Automated System is a set of drawers identified by patient room number. To access these, click on the drawers or on the **Unit Dosage** icon at the top of the screen. This provides a close-up view of the drawers. To open a drawer, click on the room number of the patient you are working with. Next, click on the medication you would like to prepare for the patient, and a label will appear, listing the medication strength, units, and dosage per unit. To exit, click **Close Drawer**; then click **View Medication Room**.

At any time, you can learn about a medication you wish to prepare for a patient by clicking on the **Drug** icon in the bottom left corner of the medication room screen or by clicking the **Drug Guide** book on the counter to the right of the unit dosage drawers. The **Drug Guide** provides information about the medications commonly included in nursing drug handbooks. Nutritional supplements and maintenance intravenous fluid preparations are not included. Highlight a medication in the alphabetical list; relevant information about the drug will appear in the screen below. To exit, click **Return to Medication Room**.

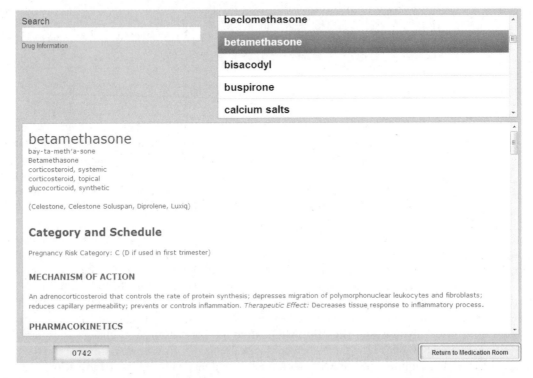

To access the MAR from the Medication Room and to review the medications ordered for a patient, click on the **MAR** icon located in the tool bar at the top of your screen and then click on the correct tab for your patient's room number. You may also click the **Review MAR** icon in the tool bar at the bottom of your screen from inside each medication storage area.

After you have chosen and prepared medications, go to the patient's room to administer them by clicking on the room number in the bottom tool bar. Inside the patient's room, click **Patient Care** and then **Medication Administration** and follow the proper administration sequence.

■ PRECEPTOR'S EVALUATIONS

When you have finished a session, click on **Leave the Floor** to go to the Floor Menu. At this point, you can click on the top icon (**Look at Your Preceptor's Evaluation**) to receive a scorecard that provides feedback on the work you completed during patient care.

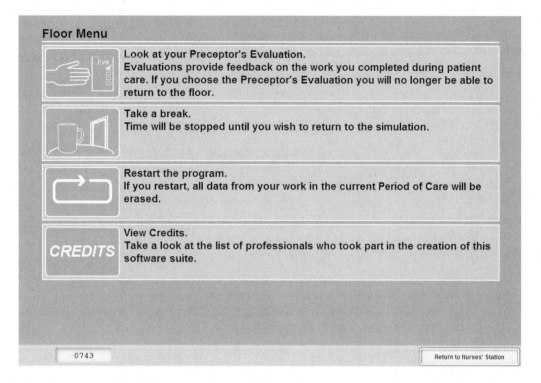

Evaluations are available for each patient you selected when you signed in for the current period of care. Click on the **Medication Scorecard** icon to see an example.

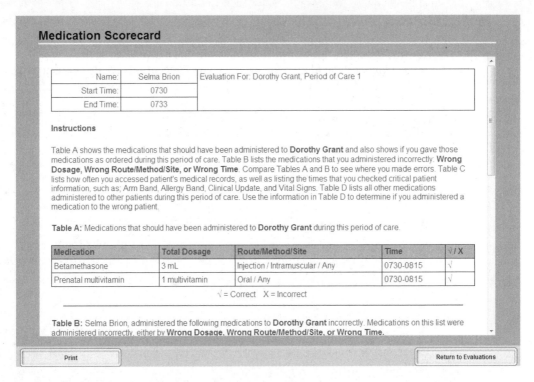

Medication Scorecard

Name:	Selma Brion	Evaluation For: Dorothy Grant, Period of Care 1
Start Time:	0730	
End Time:	0733	

Instructions

Table A shows the medications that should have been administered to **Dorothy Grant** and also shows if you gave those medications as ordered during this period of care. Table B lists the medications that you administered incorrectly: **Wrong Dosage, Wrong Route/Method/Site, or Wrong Time**. Compare Tables A and B to see where you made errors. Table C lists how often you accessed patient's medical records, as well as listing the times that you checked critical patient information, such as; Arm Band, Allergy Band, Clinical Update, and Vital Signs. Table D lists all other medications administered to other patients during this period of care. Use the information in Table D to determine if you administered a medication to the wrong patient.

Table A: Medications that should have been administered to **Dorothy Grant** during this period of care.

Medication	Total Dosage	Route/Method/Site	Time	√ / X
Betamethasone	3 mL	Injection / Intramuscular / Any	0730-0815	√
Prenatal multivitamin	1 multivitamin	Oral / Any	0730-0815	√

√ = Correct   X = Incorrect

Table B: Selma Brion, administered the following medications to **Dorothy Grant** incorrectly. Medications on this list were administered incorrectly, either by **Wrong Dosage, Wrong Route/Method/Site, or Wrong Time.**

Print   Return to Evaluations

The scorecard compares the medications you administered to a patient during a period of care with what should have been administered. Table A lists the correct medications. Table B lists any medications that were administered incorrectly.

Remember, not every medication listed on the MAR should necessarily be given. For example, a patient might have an allergy to a drug that was ordered, or a medication might have been improperly transcribed to the MAR. Predetermined medication "errors" embedded within the program challenge you to exercise critical thinking skills and professional judgment when deciding to administer a medication, just as you would in a real hospital. Use all your available resources, such as the patient's chart and the MAR, to make your decision.

Table C lists the resources that were available to assist you in medication administration. It also documents whether and when you accessed these resources. For example, did you check the patient armband or perform a check of vital signs? If so, when?

You can click **Print** to get a copy of this report if needed. When you have finished reviewing the scorecard, click **Return to Evaluations** and then **Return to Menu**.

■ FLOOR MAP

To get a general sense of your location within the hospital, you can click on the **Map** icon found in the lower right corner of most of the screens in the *Virtual Clinical Excursions—Psychiatric* program. (*Note:* If you are following this quick tour step by step, you will need to **Restart the Program** from the Floor Menu, sign in again, and go to the Nurses' Station to access the map.) When you click the **Map** icon, a floor map appears, showing the layout of the floor you are currently on, as well as a directory of the patients and services on that floor. As you move your cursor over the directory list, the location of each room is highlighted on the map (and vice versa). The floor map can be accessed from the Nurses' Station, Medication Room, and each patient's room.

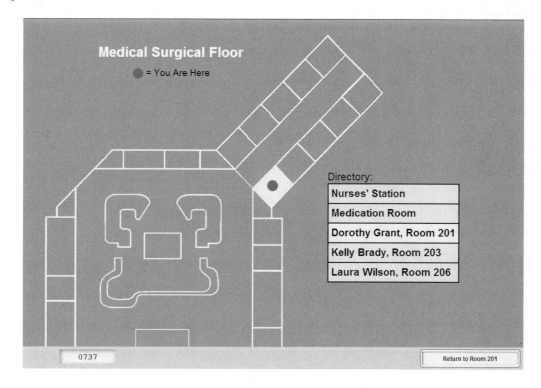

A DETAILED TOUR

If you wish to more thoroughly understand the capabilities of *Virtual Clinical Excursions—Psychiatric*, take a detailed tour by completing the following section. During this tour, we will work with a specific patient to introduce you to all the different components and learning opportunities available within the software.

■ WORKING WITH A PATIENT

Sign in and select the Obstetrics Floor for Period of Care 1 (0730-0815). From the Patient List, select Dorothy Grant in Room 201; however, do not go to the Nurses' Station yet.

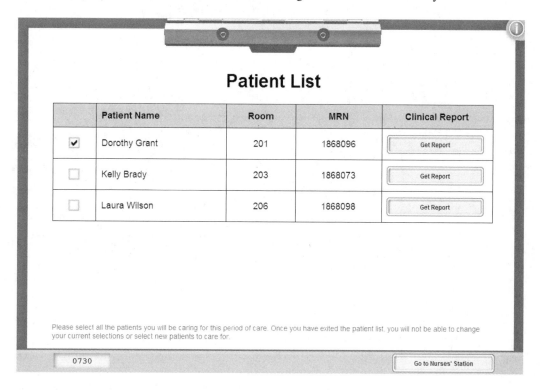

■ REPORT

In hospitals, when one shift ends and another begins, the outgoing nurse who attended a patient will give a verbal and sometimes a written summary of that patient's condition to the incoming nurse who will assume care for the patient. This summary is called a report and is an important source of data to provide an overview of a patient. Your first task is to get the clinical report on Dorothy Grant. To do this, click **Get Report** in the far right column in this patient's row. From a brief review of this summary, identify the problems and areas of concern that you will need to address for this patient.

When you have finished noting any areas of concern, click on **Go to Nurses' Station**.

■ CHARTS

You can access Dorothy Grant's chart from the Nurses' Station or from the patient's room (201). From the Nurses' Station, click on the chart rack or on the **Chart** icon in the tool bar at the top of your screen. Next, click on the chart labeled **201** to open the medical record for Dorothy Grant. Click on the **Emergency Department** tab to view a record of why this patient was admitted.

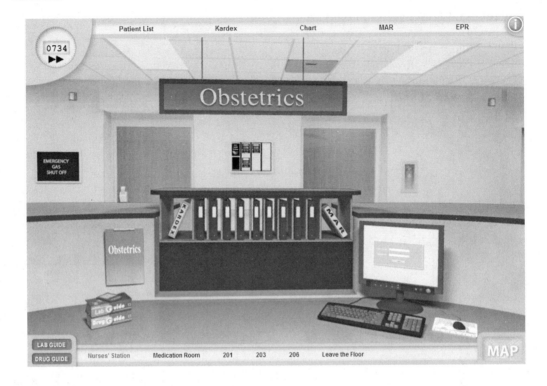

How many days has Dorothy Grant been in the hospital?

What tests were done upon her arrival in the Emergency Department and why?

What was her reason for admission?

You should also click on **Diagnostic Reports** to learn what additional tests or procedures were performed and when. Finally, review the **Nursing Admission** and **History and Physical** to learn about the health history of this patient. When you are done reviewing the chart, click **Return to Nurses' Station**.

■ MEDICATIONS

Open the Medication Administration Record (MAR) by clicking on the **MAR** icon in the tool bar at the top of your screen. *Remember:* The MAR automatically opens to the first occupied room number on the floor—which is not necessarily your patient's room number! Because you need to access Dorothy Grant's MAR, click on tab **201** (her room number). Always make sure you are giving the *Right Drug to the Right Patient!*

Examine the list of medications ordered for Dorothy Grant. In the table below, list the medications that need to be given during this period of care (0730-0815). For each medication, note the dosage, route, and time to be given.

Time	Medication	Dosage	Route

Click on **Return to Nurses' Station**. Next, click on **201** on the bottom tool bar and then verify that you are indeed in Dorothy Grant's room. Select **Clinical Alerts** (the icon to the right of Initial Observations) to check for any emerging data that might affect your medication administration priorities. Next, go to the patient's chart (click on the **Chart** icon; then click on **201**). When the chart opens, select the **Physician's Orders** tab.

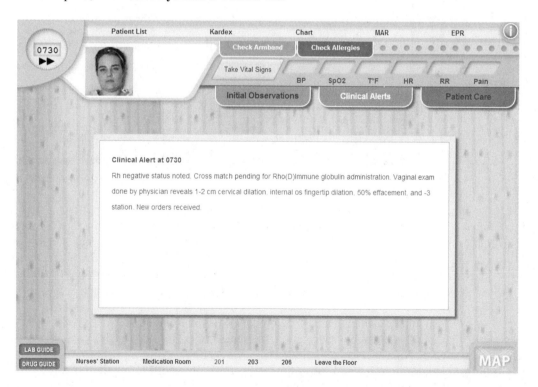

Review the orders. Have any new medications been ordered? Return to the MAR (click **Return to Room 201**; then click **MAR**). Verify that any new medications have been correctly transcribed to the MAR. Mistakes are sometimes made in the transcription process in the hospital setting, and it is sound practice to double-check any new order.

Are there any patient assessments you will need to perform before administering these medications? If so, return to Room 201 and click on **Patient Care** and then **Physical Assessment** to complete those assessments before proceeding.

Now click on the **Medication Room** icon in the tool bar at the bottom of your screen to locate and prepare the medications for Dorothy Grant.

In the Medication Room, you must access the medications for Dorothy Grant from the specific dispensing system in which each medication is stored. Locate each medication that needs to be given in this time period and click on **Put Medication on Tray** as appropriate. (*Hint:* Look in **Unit Dosage** drawer first.) When you are finished, click on **Close Drawer** and then on **View Medication Room**. Now click on the medication tray on the counter on the left side of the medication room screen to begin preparing the medications you have selected. (*Remember:* You can also click **Preparation** in the tool bar at the top of the screen.)

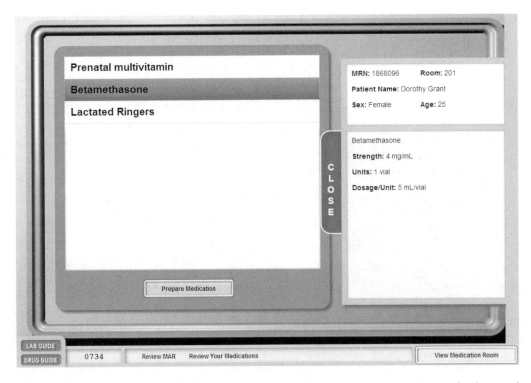

In the preparation area, you should see a list of the medications you put on the tray in the previous steps. Click on the first medication and then click **Prepare**. Follow the onscreen instructions of the Preparation Wizard, providing any data requested. As an example, let's follow the preparation process for betamethasone, one of the medications due to be administered to Dorothy Grant during this period of care. To begin, click to select **Betamethasone**; then click **Prepare**. Now work through the Preparation Wizard sequence as detailed below:

Amount of medication in the ampule: Betamethasone 5 mL.
Enter the amount of medication you will draw up into a syringe: **3 mL**.
Click **Next**.
Select the patient to receive the medication: **Room 201, Dorothy Grant**.
Click **Finish**.
Click **Return to Medication Room**.

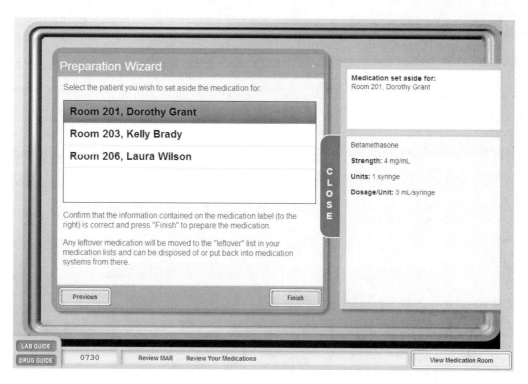

Follow this same basic process for the other medications due to be administered to Dorothy Grant during this period of care. (*Hint:* Look in **IV Storage** and **Automated System**.)

PREPARATION WIZARD EXCEPTIONS

- Some medications in *Virtual Clinical Excursions—Psychiatric* are prepared by the pharmacy (e.g., IV antibiotics) and taken to the patient room as a whole. This is common practice in most hospitals.
- Blood products are not administered by students through the *Virtual Clinical Excursions—Psychiatric* simulations because blood administration follows specific protocols not covered in this program.
- The *Virtual Clinical Excursions—Psychiatric* simulations do not allow for mixing more than one type of medication, such as regular and Lente insulins, in the same syringe. In the clinical setting, when multiple types of insulin are ordered for a patient, the regular insulin is drawn up first, followed by the longer-acting insulin. Insulin is always administered in a special unit-marked syringe.

Now return to Room 201 (click on **201** on the bottom tool bar) to administer Dorothy Grant's medications.

At any time during the medication administration process, you can perform a further review of systems, take vital signs, check information contained within the chart, or verify patient identity and allergies. Inside Dorothy Grant's room, click **Take Vital Signs**. (*Note:* These findings change over time to reflect the temporal changes you would find in a patient similar to Dorothy Grant.)

When you have gathered all the data you need, click on **Patient Care** and then select **Medication Administration**. Any medications you prepared in the previous steps should be listed on the left side of your screen. Let's continue the administration process with the betamethasone ordered for Dorothy Grant. Click to highlight **Betamethasone** in the list of medications. Next, click on the down arrow to the right of **Select** and choose **Administer** from the drop-down menu. This will activate the Administration Wizard. Complete the Wizard sequence as follows:

- Route: **Injection**
- Method: **Intramuscular**
- Site: **Any** (choose one)
- Click **Administer to Patient** arrow.
- Would you like to document this administration in the MAR? **Yes**
- Click **Finish** arrow.

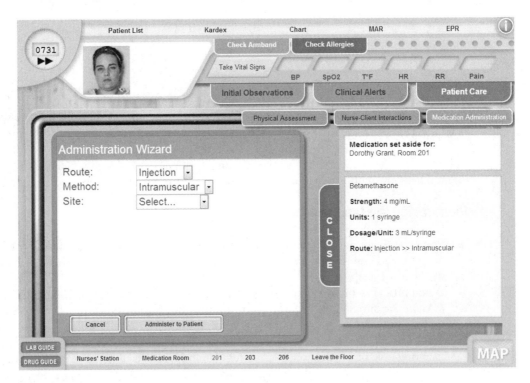

Your selections are recorded by a tracking system and evaluated on a Medication Scorecard stored under Preceptor's Evaluations. This scorecard can be viewed, printed, and given to your instructor. To access the Preceptor's Evaluations, click on **Leave the Floor**. When the Floor Menu appears, select **Look at Your Preceptor's Evaluation**. Then click on **Medication Scorecard** inside the box with Dorothy Grant's name (see example on the following page).

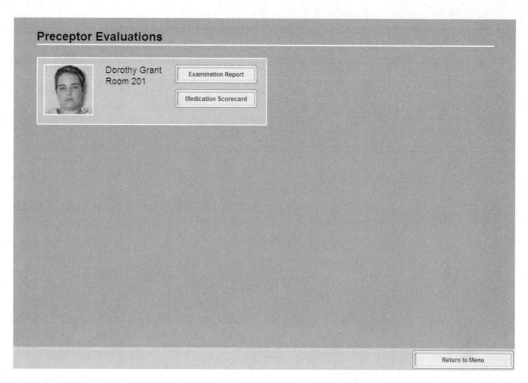

■ MEDICATION SCORECARD

- First, review Table A. Was betamethasone given correctly? Did you give the other medications as ordered?
- Table B shows you which (if any) medications you gave incorrectly.
- Table C addresses the resources used for Dorothy Grant. Did you access the patient's chart, MAR, EPR, or Kardex as needed to make safe medication administration decisions?
- Did you check the patient's armband to verify her identity? Did you check whether your patient had any known allergies to medications? Were vital signs taken?

When you have finished reviewing the scorecard, click **Return to Evaluations** and then **Return to Menu**.

■ **VITAL SIGNS**

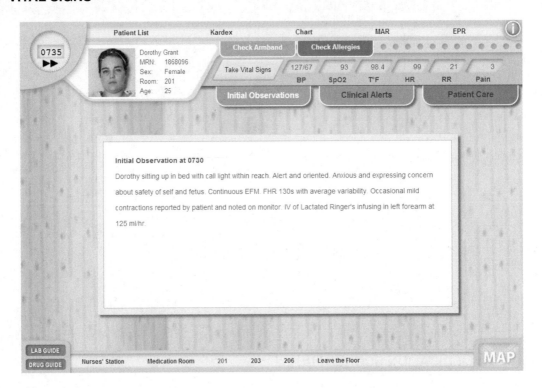

Vital signs, often considered the traditional "signs of life," include body temperature, heart rate, respiratory rate, blood pressure, oxygen saturation of the blood, and pain level.

Inside Dorothy Grant's room, click **Take Vital Signs**. (*Note:* If you are following this detailed tour step by step, you will need to **Restart the Program** from the Floor Menu, sign in again for Period of Care 1, and navigate to Room 201.) Collect vital signs for this patient and record them below. Note the time at which you collected each of these data. (*Remember:* You can take vital signs at any time. The data change over time to reflect the temporal changes you would find in a patient similar to Dorothy Grant.)

Vital Signs	Findings/Time
Blood pressure	
O$_2$ saturation	
Temperature	
Heart rate	
Respiratory rate	
Pain rating	

After you are done, click on the **EPR** icon located in the tool bar at the top of the screen. Your username and password are automatically provided. Click on **Login** to enter the EPR. To access Dorothy Grant's records, click on the down arrow next to Patient and choose her room number, **201**. Select **Vital Signs** as the category. Next, in the empty time column on the far right, record the vital signs data you just collected in Dorothy Grant's room. If you need help with this process, refer to the Electronic Patient Record (EPR) section of the Quick Tour. Now compare these findings with the data you collected earlier for this patient's vital signs. Use these earlier findings to establish a baseline for each of the vital signs.

    a.   Are any of the data you collected significantly different from the baseline for a particular vital sign?

        Circle One: Yes   No

    b.   If "Yes," which data are different?

■ PHYSICAL ASSESSMENT

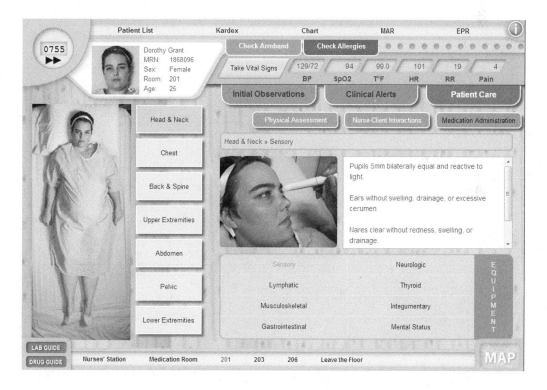

After you have finished examining the EPR for vital signs, click **Exit EPR** to return to Room 201. Click **Patient Care** and then **Physical Assessment**. Think about the information you received in the report at the beginning of this shift, as well as what you may have learned about this patient from the chart. Based on this, what area(s) of examination should you pay most attention to at this time? Is there any equipment you should be monitoring? Conduct a physical assessment of the body areas and systems that you consider priorities for Dorothy Grant. For example, select **Head & Neck**; then click on and assess **Sensory** and **Lymphatic**. Complete any other assessment(s) you think are necessary at this time. In the following table, record the data you collected during this examination.

Area of Examination	Findings
Head & Neck Sensory	
Head & Neck Lymphatic	

After you have finished collecting these data, return to the EPR. Compare the data that were already in the record with those you just collected.

a. Are any of the data you collected significantly different from the baselines for this patient?

   Circle One: Yes   No

b. If "Yes," which data are different?

◼ NURSE-CLIENT INTERACTIONS

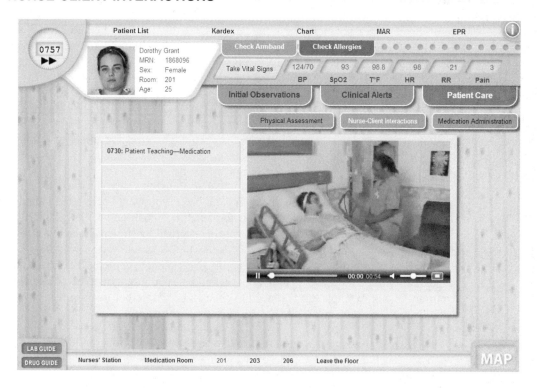

Click on **Patient Care** from inside Dorothy Grant's room (201). Now click on **Nurse-Client Interactions** to access a short video titled **Patient Teaching—Medication**, which is available for viewing at or after 0730 (based on the virtual clock in the upper left corner of your screen; see *Note* below). To begin the video, click on the white arrow next to its title. You will observe a nurse communicating with Dorothy Grant. There are many variations of nursing practice, some exemplifying "best" practice and some not. Note whether the nurse in this interaction displays professional behavior and compassionate care. Are her words congruent with what is going on with the patient? Does this interaction "feel right" to you? If not, how would you handle this situation differently? Explain.

Note: If the video you wish to view is not listed, this means you have not yet reached the correct virtual time to view that video. Check the virtual clock; you may return to access the video once its designated time has occurred—as long as you do so within the same period of care. Or you can click on the fast-forward icon within the virtual clock to advance the time by 2-minute intervals. You will then need to click again on **Patient Care** and **Nurse-Client Interactions** to refresh the screen.

At least one Nurse-Client Interactions video is available during each period of care. Viewing these videos can help you learn more about what is occurring with a patient at a certain time and also prompt you to discern between nurse communications that are ideal and those that need improvement. Compassionate care and the ability to communicate clearly are essential components of delivering quality nursing care, and it is during your clinical time that you will begin to refine these skills.

■ **COLLECTING AND EVALUATING DATA**

Each of the activities you perform in the Patient Care environment generates a significant amount of assessment data. Remember that after you collect data, you can record your findings in the EPR. You can also review the EPR, patient's chart, videos, and MAR at any time. You will get plenty of practice collecting and then evaluating data in context of the patient's course.

Now, here's an important question for you:

> Did the previous sequence of exercises provide the most efficient way to assess Dorothy Grant?

For example, you went to the patient's room to get vital signs, then back to the EPR to enter data and compare your findings with extant data. Next, you went back to the patient's room to do a physical examination, then again back to the EPR to enter and review data. If this back-and-forth process of data collection and recording seemed inefficient, remember the following:

- Plan all of your nursing activities to maximize efficiency, while at the same time optimizing the quality of patient care. (Think about what data you might need before performing certain tasks. For example, do you need to check a heart rate before administering a cardiac medication or check an IV site before starting an infusion?)

- You collect a tremendous amount of data when you work with a patient. Very few people can accurately remember all these data for more than a few minutes. Develop efficient assessment skills, and record data as soon as possible after collecting them.

- Assessment data are only the starting point for the nursing process.

Make a clear distinction between these first exercises and how you actually provide nursing care. These initial exercises were designed to involve you actively in the use of different software components. This workbook focuses on sensible practices for implementing the nursing process in ways that ensure the highest-quality care of patients.

Most important, remember that a human being changes through time, and that these changes include both the physical and psychosocial facets of a person as a living organism. Think about this for a moment. Some patients may change physically in a very short time (a patient with emerging myocardial infarction) or more slowly (a patient with a chronic illness). Patients' overall physical and psychosocial conditions may improve or deteriorate. They may have effective coping skills and familial support, or they may feel alone and full of despair. In fact, each individual is a complex mix of physical and psychosocial elements, and at least some of these elements usually change through time.

Thus it is crucial that you *DO NOT* think of the nursing process as a simple one-time, five-step procedure consisting of assessment, nursing diagnosis, planning, implementation, and evaluation. Rather, the nursing process should be utilized as a creative and systematic approach to delivering nursing care. Furthermore, because all living organisms are constantly changing, we must apply the nursing process over and over. Each time we follow the nursing process for an individual patient, we refine our understanding of that patient's physical and psychosocial conditions based on collection and analysis of many different types of data. *Virtual Clinical Excursions—Psychiatric* will help you develop both the creativity and the systematic approach needed to become a nurse who is equipped to deliver the highest-quality care to all patients.

REDUCING MEDICATION ERRORS

Earlier in the detailed tour, you learned the basic steps of medication preparation and administration. The following simulations will allow you to practice those skills further—with an increased emphasis on reducing medication errors by using the Medication Scorecard to evaluate your work.

Sign in to work on the Obstetrics Floor at Pacific View Regional Hospital for Period of Care 1. (*Note:* If you are already working with another patient or during another period of care, click on **Leave the Floor** and then **Restart the Program**; then sign in.)

From the Patient List, select Dorothy Grant. Then click on **Go to Nurses' Station**. Complete the following steps to prepare and administer medications to Dorothy Grant.

- Click on **Medication Room** on the tool bar at the bottom of your screen.
- Click on **MAR** and then on tab **201** to determine medications that have been ordered for Dorothy Grant. (*Note:* You may click on **Review MAR** at any time to verify the correct medication order. Always remember to check the patient name on the MAR to make sure you have the correct patient's record. You must click on the correct room number tab within the MAR.) Click on **Return to Medication Room** after reviewing the correct MAR.
- Click on **Unit Dosage** (or on the Unit Dosage cabinet); from the close-up view, click on drawer **201**.
- Select the medications you would like to administer. After each selection, click **Put Medication on Tray**. When you are finished selecting medications, click **Close Drawer** and then **View Medication Room**.
- Click **Automated System** (or on the Automated System unit itself). Click **Login**.
- On the next screen, specify the correct patient and drawer location.
- Select the medication you would like to administer and click **Put Medication on Tray**. Repeat this process if you wish to administer other medications from the Automated System.
- When you are finished, click **Close Drawer** and **View Medication Room**.
- From the Medication Room, click **Preparation** (or on the preparation tray).
- From the list of medications on your tray, highlight the correct medication to administer and click **Prepare**.
- This activates the Preparation Wizard. Supply any requested information; then click **Next**.
- Now select the correct patient to receive this medication and click **Finish**.
- Repeat the previous three steps until all medications that you want to administer are prepared.
- You can click on **Review Your Medications** and then on **Return to Medication Room** when ready. Once you are back in the Medication Room, go directly to Dorothy Grant's room by clicking on **201** at the bottom of the screen.
- Inside the patient's room, administer the medication, utilizing the six rights of medication administration. After you have collected the appropriate assessment data and are ready for administration, click **Patient Care** and then **Medication Administration**. Verify that the correct patient and medication(s) appear in the left-hand window. Highlight the first medication you wish to administer; then click the down arrow next to Select. From the drop-down menu, select **Administer** and complete the Administration Wizard by providing any information requested. When the Wizard stops asking for information, click **Administer to Patient**. Specify **Yes** when asked whether this administration should be recorded in the MAR. Finally, click **Finish**.

■ **SELF-EVALUATION**

Now let's see how you did during your medication administration!

- Click on **Leave the Floor** at the bottom of your screen. From the Floor Menu, select **Look at Your Preceptor's Evaluation**. Then click **Medication Scorecard**.

The following exercises will help you identify medication errors, investigate possible reasons for these errors, and reduce or prevent medication errors in the future.

1. Start by examining Table A. These are the medications you should have given to Dorothy Grant during this period of care. If each of the medications in Table A has a ✓ by it, then you made no errors. Congratulations!

If any medication has an X by it, then you made one or more medication errors.

Compare Tables A and B to determine which of the following types of errors you made: Wrong Dose, Wrong Route/Method/Site, or Wrong Time. Follow these steps:
   a. Find medications in Table A that were given incorrectly.
   b. Now see if those same medications are in Table B, which shows what you actually administered to Dorothy Grant.
   c. Comparing Tables A and B, match the Strength, Dose, Route/Method/Site, and Time for each medication you administered incorrectly.
   d. Then, using the form below, list the medications given incorrectly and mark the errors you made for each medication.

Medication	Strength	Dosage	Route	Method	Site	Time
	❑	❑	❑	❑	❑	❑
	❑	❑	❑	❑	❑	❑
	❑	❑	❑	❑	❑	❑
	❑	❑	❑	❑	❑	❑

2. To help you reduce future medication errors, consider the following list of possible reasons for errors.

- Did not check drug against MAR for correct medication, correct dose, correct patient, correct route, correct time, correct documentation.
- Did not check drug dose against MAR three times.
- Did not open the unit dose package in the patient's room.
- Did not correctly identify the patient using two identifiers.
- Did not administer the drug on time.
- Did not verify patient allergies.
- Did not check the patient's current condition or vital sign parameters.
- Did not consider why the patient would be receiving this drug.
- Did not question why the drug was in the patient's drawer.
- Did not check the physician's order and/or check with the pharmacist when there was a question about the drug or dose.
- Did not verify that no adverse effects had occurred from a previous dose.

Based on the list of possibilities you just reviewed, determine how you made each error and record the reason in the form below:

Medication	Reason for Error

3. Look again at Table B. Are there medications listed that are not in Table A? If so, you gave a medication to Dorothy Grant that she should not have received. Complete the following exercises to help you understand how such an error might have been made.

    a. Perhaps you gave a medication that was on Dorothy Grant's MAR for this period of care, without recognizing that a change had occurred in the patient's condition, which should have caused you to reconsider. Review patient records as necessary and complete the following form:

Medication	Possible Reasons Not to Give This Medication

    b. Another possibility is that you gave Dorothy Grant a medication that should have been given at a different time. Check her MAR and complete the form below to determine whether you made a Wrong Time error:

Medication	Given to Dorothy Grant at What Time	Should Have Been Given at What Time

c. Maybe you gave another patient's medication to Dorothy Grant. In this case, you made a Wrong Patient error. Check the MARs of other patients and use the form below to determine whether you made this type of error:

Medication	Given to Dorothy Grant	Should Have Been Given to

4. The Medication Scorecard provides some other interesting sources of information. For example, if there is a medication selected for Dorothy Grant but it was not given to her, there will be an X by that medication in Table A, but it will not appear in Table B. In that case, you might have given this medication to some other patient, which is another type of Wrong Patient error. To investigate further, look at Table D, which lists the medications you gave to other patients. See whether you can find any medications ordered for Dorothy Grant that were given to another patient by mistake. However, before you make any decisions, be sure to cross-check the MAR for other patients because the same medication may have been ordered for multiple patients. Use the following form to record your findings:

Medication	Should Have Been Given to Dorothy Grant	Given by Mistake to

5. Now take some time to review the medication exercises you just completed. Use the form below to create an overall analysis of what you have learned. Once again, record each of the medication errors you made, including the type of each error. Then, for each error you made, indicate specifically what you would do differently to prevent this type of error from occurring again.

Medication	Type of Error	Error Prevention Tactic

Submit this form to your instructor if required as a graded assignment, or simply use these exercises to improve your understanding of medication errors and how to reduce them.

Name: _____   Date: _____

Mental Health and Mental Illness

Reading Assignments:
  Halter: Varcarolis' Foundations of Psychiatric Mental Health Nursing, 7th edition
       (Chapters 1, 4, and 7)
  Keltner: Psychiatric Nursing, 7th edition (Chapters 1-6)
  Varcarolis: Essentials of Psychiatric Mental Health Nursing, 2nd edition Revised Reprint
       (Chapter 2)

Patient: Harry George, Medical-Surgical Floor, Room 401

Goal: To understand the role of the nurse in caring for a patient along the mental health and mental illness
   continuum.

Objectives:

- Define mental health.
- Discuss the concepts of the mental health and mental illness continuum.
- Understand the role of the nurse in caring for a patient along the mental health and mental
  illness continuum.
- Identify effective communication techniques used by the nurse in nurse-patient interactions.
- Compare and contrast the therapeutic care for a patient in the hospital and in the community.

Exercise 1

Writing Activity

30 minutes

1. Provide a definition of mental health that includes at least four defining characteristics.

2. Which statements are true regarding the concepts of mental health and mental illness? Select all that apply.

   _____ Many forms of unusual behavior may be tolerated, depending on the cultural norms.

   _____ Mentally ill individuals are those who violate social norms.

   _____ There are many influences that impact the mental health of an individual, such as heredity, culture, health practices, support, life stressors, and biological disorders.

   _____ Mental illness is defined as being different or strange.

   _____ Mental health means one is logical and rational.

   _____ All human behavior lies somewhere along a continuum of mental health and mental illness.

3. Discuss the term *resilience* as it relates to mental health.

4. Describe effective characteristics of therapeutic communication related to the nurse-patient relationship.

5. Describe the goals of a nurse working with a patient across the continuum of care from an acute care hospital setting to a community-based setting.

Setting	Nurse-Patient Relationship Goals
Acute care hospital setting	
Community-based setting	

Exercise 2

Virtual Hospital Activity

30 minutes

- Sign in to work at Pacific View Regional Hospital on the Medical-Surgical Floor for Period of Care 1. (*Note:* If you are already in the virtual hospital from a previous exercise, click on **Leave the Floor** and then **Restart the Program** to get to the sign-in window.)
- From the Patient List, select Harry George (Room 401).
- Click on **Go to Nurses' Station**.
- Click on **Chart** and then on **401**.
- Read the **History and Physical**.
- Next, read the **Nursing Admission**.

1. What stressor(s) contributed to Harry George's current life situation?
   a. Motorcycle accident
   b. Chronic left foot bone infection and severe pain
   c. Estrangement from wife and two sons
   d. Loss of job
   e. Homelessness
   f. All of the above

2. After reviewing the History and Physical and the Nursing Admission, list Harry George's medical diagnoses below. For each diagnosis, identify potential nursing problems associated with that diagnosis.

Medical Diagnoses   **Nursing Problems**

3. Match each type of health education intervention with the specific health topics Harry George will need during hospitalization and after discharge.

Type of Health Education Intervention

_____ Increase awareness of issues related to health and illness

_____ Increase understanding of potential stressors, possible outcomes, and alternative coping responses

_____ Increase knowledge of where and how to obtain resources

_____ Increase actual abilities

Specific Health Topic

a. Developing healthy coping skills (such as stress reduction), developing motivation and self-esteem, problem solving, and stress management

b. Learning how to become clean and sober, caring for self, managing pain and diabetes, and smoking cessation

c. Finding housing, finding/keeping job, and locating family members

d. Dealing with loss of family and job, homelessness, and pain

4. How important is pain management in Harry George's rehabilitation and recovery?

5. In view of Harry George's current living situation and 4-year history of alcoholism, what do you think would be the best type of program to help him quit drinking upon discharge?
   a. Community-based sober living house
   b. Inpatient alcohol/drug treatment program
   c. Outpatient visits with a drug/alcohol counselor
   d. Does not really matter because he will not stop drinking

6. Below and on the next page, describe the challenges that Harry George faces in his recovery in the following areas.

Area of Rehabilitation/Recovery	Challenge
Activities of daily living (ADL)	
Interpersonal relationships	
Self-esteem	
Motivation	
Illness management	

Area of Rehabilitation/Recovery	Challenge
Strengths	

7. What hospital-based resources does the nurse have available to help Harry George with the community needs he will have after discharge?

8. Using information from your textbook and taking into consideration Harry George's history and current needs, discuss how a positive change in his living/social environment could affect his rehabilitation and recovery.

Cultural Competence Related to Mental Health Nursing

Reading Assignments:

Halter: Varcarolis' Foundations of Psychiatric Mental Health Nursing, 7th edition
(Chapters 5 and 7)

Keltner: Psychiatric Nursing, 7th edition (Chapters 14 and 15)

Varcarolis: Essentials of Psychiatric Mental Health Nursing, 2nd edition Revised Reprint
(Chapters 7, 8, and 9)

Patient: Carlos Reyes, Skilled Nursing Floor, Room 504

Goal: To understand cultural aspects of psychiatric nursing care.

Objectives:

- Understand how culture helps define mental health and mental illness.
- Define culturally competent care.
- Define practice barriers to providing culturally competent care.
- Describe methods the nurse can use to overcome barriers to culturally competent care.
- Describe methods the nurse can use to provide culturally competent care.
- Identify the basic elements in a cultural assessment.
- Understand the role language and culture play in the assessment, diagnosis, and treatment of mental illness.
- Describe the importance of including assessment of spirituality in the plan of psychiatric nursing care.

Exercise 1

Writing Activity

15 minutes

1. Place an X next to each true statement regarding culture and mental health and mental illness. Select all that apply.

   __X__ Each cultural group has cultural beliefs, values, and practices that guide its members in ways of thinking and acting.

   __X__ The framework that describes mental health and illness in the United States is based on Eastern thought.

   _____ Culture defines the differences between mental health and mental illness.

   __X__ Deviance from cultural expectations is considered to be a problem and is usually seen by the cultural group as an "illness."

   _____ The same thoughts and behaviors that are considered mental health in one culture can be considered an illness in another culture.

2. In providing care to culturally diverse populations, the nurse will encounter barriers in practice and must be knowledgeable about methods to overcome these barriers. Listed below and on the next page are three practice issues and their associated difficulties. Complete the table by listing ways the nurse can overcome each barrier.

Cultural Practice Issue	Barrier	Examples for Overcoming Barrier
Communication	Miscommunication because of differences in spoken language and in the meaning of nonverbal communication	
Assessment	Failure to assess the patient's cultural perspective using available clinical cultural assessment tools	

Cultural Practice Issue	Barrier	Examples for Overcoming Barrier
Values and beliefs	Lack of knowledge and sensitivity regarding the patient's beliefs and practices; patient may be unaware of the nurse's cultural perspective	
Ethnopharmacology	Genetic variations in drug metabolism found in people of all ethnicities	

3. List the basic elements that nurses must include in their cultural assessment of a patient that may be needed to meet the cultural beliefs and practices, needs, and preferences.

4. Using the process of cultural competence in delivering mental health care, describe how the psychiatric mental health nurse can develop culturally competent care in the following areas.

Area	Nurse's Behavior
Cultural awareness	
Cultural knowledge	
Cultural encounters	
Cultural skill	
Cultural desire	

Exercise 2

Virtual Hospital Activity

45 minutes

- Sign in to work at Pacific View Regional Hospital on the Skilled Nursing Floor for Period of Care 1. (*Note:* If you are already in the virtual hospital from a previous exercise, click on **Leave the Floor** and then **Restart the Program** to get to the sign-in window.)
- From the Patient List, select Carlos Reyes (Room 504).
- Click on **Go to Nurses' Station**.
- Click on **Chart** and then on **504**.
- Read the **History and Physical** and **Nursing Admission** records.

1. According to the medical record, Carlos Reyes' cultural background is

   _____.

2. What are some characteristics of the culture you identified in question 1?

   - patient assessment (initiating communication)

   * nurse reassess patients medications due to lethargy

   - Patient teaching to the family Family teaching about the effects of the drug
   - nurse agreed to withold medication as per

3. What are the cultural factors to consider in providing nursing care for Carlos Reyes? sons request; hold am dose.

- Click on **Return to Nurses' Station**.
- Click on **504** at the bottom of the screen.
- Click on **Patient Care** and then on **Nurse-Client Interactions**.
- To answer questions 4-8, you will need to select and view the video titles listed below.
  (*Note:* Check the virtual clock to see whether enough time has elapsed. You can use the fast-forward feature to advance the time by 2-minute intervals if the video is not yet available. Then click on **Patient Care** and **Nurse-Client Interactions** to refresh the screen.)
  - 0740: Family Teaching—Medication
  - 0745: Drowsiness—Contributing Factor
  - 0750: Assessment—Level of Assistance
- After viewing the above three videos, click on the **Drug** icon in the lower left corner of your screen. Use the Search box or the scroll bar to find information on oxazepam.

4. What two interventions did the nurse implement to address Carlos Reyes' son's concerns about his father's drowsiness?

5. What other actions could the nurse have taken?

6. Explain the indication for oxazepam and the effect it has on brain function. Identify the side effect that was concerning Carlos Reyes' son.

7. What aspects of the mental status exam is the nurse attempting to assess?
   a. Appearance, speech, motor activity, and interaction
   b. Level of consciousness
   c. Emotional state: mood and affect
   d. All of the above

8. What level of assistance will Carlos Reyes need in order to sit up and eat his breakfast? Discuss the role of his family at mealtime.

The Nurse-Patient Relationship

Reading Assignments:

Halter: Varcarolis' Foundations of Psychiatric Mental Health Nursing, 7th edition (Chapter 8)

Keltner: Psychiatric Nursing, 7th edition (Chapters 6 and 7)

Varcarolis: Essentials of Psychiatric Mental Health Nursing, 2nd edition Revised Reprint (Chapter 9)

Patients: Jacquline Catanazaro, Medical-Surgical Floor, Room 402

Kathryn Doyle, Skilled Nursing Floor, Room 503

Goal: To learn the importance of the therapeutic nurse-patient relationship and be able to apply therapeutic communication techniques with patients.

Objectives:

- List the characteristics and goals of the therapeutic nurse-patient relationship.
- Identify the personal qualities of the nurse that are necessary to communicate effectively.
- Describe the qualities of genuineness, empathy, and positive regard in the therapeutic nurse-patient relationship.
- Discuss the verbal and nonverbal components of communication.
- Identify the types of boundary issues and their importance in the nurse-patient relationship.
- Identify transference and countertransference in the therapeutic nurse-patient relationship.
- Describe the phases of a therapeutic nurse-patient relationship.
- Evaluate effective communication techniques used by the nurse in nurse-patient interactions.

Exercise 1

Writing Activity

30 minutes

1. Health care has increasingly embraced the concept of patient-centered care. That includes dignity and respect, sharing of information, patient and family participation, and collaboration with providers. Patient-centered care is the therapeutic nurse-patient relationship. Below, list four characteristics and four goals of the therapeutic relationship.

Characteristics of a Therapeutic Relationship	Goals of a Therapeutic Relationship
(1) Therapeutic Communication	(1) Facilitet verbal expression of distressing thoughts/ feelings.
(2) Client- centered care	(2) Assist p'ls to develope self- awareness + insignt into their thoughts, feelings, + behaviours in order for them to better manage ADLs.
(3) Maintaining boundaries	(3) helping patients examine self-defeating behaviours + test alternatives.
(4) protecting the client from abuse	(4) promote self-care + independence

2. Which personal behaviors, qualities, and skills must the nurse have in order to communicate therapeutically with patients? Select all that apply.

  _X_ Accountability

  _X_ Focus on the patient's needs

  _X_ Clinical competence

  _X_ Delaying judgment

  _____ Self-awareness

  _____ Understanding of one's own values and beliefs

3. Discuss communication and the importance of its verbal and nonverbal components.

> central to the formation of the therapeutic relationship
> both forms of communication are essential for conveying an idea or message as well as the intent behind it as 90% of communication is interpretted via non-verbal ques.

4. Therapeutic listening, an important component of the therapeutic use of self, is composed of which attributes? Select all that apply.

____X____ Using eye contact

____X____ Being relaxed

____X____ Being patient

_____ Asking questions

?. ____X____ Offering empathy and support

____X____ Summarizing important points

_____ Looking away often to appear detached

____X____ Responding verbally and nonverbally to encourage patient to continue

_____ Sitting in a closed position

5. Describe the personal qualities of genuineness, positive regard (respect), and empathy that a nurse must have in order to establish and maintain a therapeutic relationship.

Genuineness

 ↳ Self-awareness of ones feelings as they arise w/i relationship + ability to communicate them when appropriate

 ↳ gives sense that outward presentation is congruent w/ internal process - helps build trust
 ↳ Conveyed by listening to + communicating w/ pts w/o distorting their msg.

Positive regard (respect)

 ↳ ability to view another as worthy of being cared for about + as someone who has strengths + achievement potential

 ↳ conveyed indirectly by attitude/action

Empathy

 ↳ understanding the world from the patients perspective - remaining unjudgmental + uncritical

 ↳ involves
   1) Accurately perceiving pts situation, perspective, feeling.
   2) Communicating ones understanding to the pt + checking for accuracy
   3) Acting on this understanding.

6. Establishing and maintaining boundaries in the nurse-patient relationship are challenging tasks. Boundaries are always at risk for being blurred. What are two common circumstances that can produce blurring of boundaries?

   1) When the relationship is allowed to slip into a social context

   2) When the psychiatric nurses needs (for attention, affection, emotional support) are met at the expense of the patients needs.

7. Role blurring is often the result of unrecognized transference or countertransference. Match each term with its definition.

Term	Definition
_B_ Countertransference	a. Unconscious response in which the patient experiences feelings and attitudes toward the nurse originally associated with other significant figures in the patient's life.
_A_ Transference	b. Response used by the nurse; the specific emotional response to the qualities of the patient. This is inappropriate to the content and context of the therapeutic relationship.

8. Identify the three phases of the nurse-patient relationship by matching each phase with its characteristics.

Phase	Characteristics
_B_ Orientation	a. Signifies a loss for both the patient and nurse; goals and objectives are summarized, and progress is reviewed; possible regression.
_C_ Working	b. Trust is established, relationship is defined, contracts are established, and confidentiality and termination are discussed.
_A_ Termination	c. Focus is on maintenance, gathering more information, promoting patient's strengths, facilitating behavioral change, overcoming resistance, evaluating problems and goals, and promoting practice and expression of alternative adaptive behaviors.

Exercise 2

Virtual Hospital Activity

30 minutes

- Sign in to work at Pacific View Regional Hospital on the Medical-Surgical Floor for Period of Care 1. (*Note:* If you are already in the virtual hospital from a previous exercise, click on **Leave the Floor** and then **Restart the Program** to get to the sign-in window.)
- From the Patient List, select Jacquline Catanazaro (Room 402).
- Click on **Go to Nurses' Station** and then on **402** at the bottom of the screen.
- Click on **Patient Care** and then on **Nurse-Client Interactions**.
- Select and view the video titled **0730: Intervention—Airway**. (*Note:* Check the virtual clock to see whether enough time has elapsed. You can use the fast-forward feature to advance the time by 2-minute intervals if the video is not yet available. Then click on **Patient Care** and **Nurse-Client Interactions** to refresh the screen.)

1. As you observe the 0730 video, make note of the therapeutic verbal and nonverbal communication techniques the nurse uses. Record these in the first column of the table below. Then, for each technique you identify, list specific examples of verbal and nonverbal communication used by the nurse that demonstrate the technique.

Therapeutic Communication Techniques Used by Nurse	Specific Examples of Nurse Communication

Verbal

Clarifying —

Validating —

Clinical Competence

Nonverbal

leaning towards pt

eye contact

Therapeutic touch

Now let's jump ahead in time to observe a later interaction between the nurse and this patient.

- Click on **Leave the Floor** and then on **Restart the Program**.
- Sign in to work on the Medical-Surgical Floor for Period of Care 2.
- From the Patient List, select Jacquline Catanazaro (Room 402).
- Click on **Go to Nurses' Station** and then on **402** at the bottom of the screen.
- Click on **Patient Care** and then on **Nurse-Client Interactions**.
- Select and view the video titled **1115: Assessment—Readiness to Learn**. (*Note:* Check the virtual clock to see whether enough time has elapsed. You can use the fast-forward feature to advance the time by 2-minute intervals if the video is not yet available. Then click on **Patient Care** and **Nurse-Client Interactions** to refresh the screen.)

2. As you observe the 1115 video, make note of the therapeutic verbal and nonverbal communication techniques the nurse uses. Record these in the first column of the table below. Then, for each technique you identify, list specific examples of verbal and nonverbal communication used by the nurse that demonstrate the technique.

Therapeutic Communication Techniques Used by Nurse	Specific Examples of Nurse Communication
Verbal	
Nonverbal	

Next, let's look at an interaction between the nurse and a different patient.

- Click on **Leave the Floor** and then on **Restart the Program**.
- Sign in to work on the Skilled Nursing Floor for Period of Care 1.
- From the Patient List, select Kathryn Doyle (Room 503).
- Click on **Go to Nurses' Station** and then on **503** at the bottom of the screen.
- Click on **Patient Care** and then on **Nurse-Client Interactions**.
- Select and view the video titled **0730: Assessment—Biopsychosocial**. (*Note:* Check the virtual clock to see whether enough time has elapsed. You can use the fast-forward feature to advance the time by 2-minute intervals if the video is not yet available. Then click on **Patient Care** and **Nurse-Client Interactions** to refresh the screen.)

3. As you observe the 0730 video, make note of the therapeutic verbal and nonverbal communication techniques the nurse uses. Record these in the first column of the table below. Then, for each technique you identify, list specific examples of verbal and nonverbal communication used by the nurse that demonstrate the technique.

Therapeutic Communication Techniques Used by Nurse	Specific Examples of Nurse Communication
Verbal	
Nonverbal	

Stress

Reading Assignments:

Halter: Varcarolis' Foundations of Psychiatric Mental Health Nursing, 7th edition (Chapter 10)

Keltner: Psychiatric Nursing, 7th edition (Chapters 9 and 27)

Varcarolis: Essentials of Psychiatric Mental Health Nursing, 2nd edition Revised Reprint (Chapter 10)

Patient: Kelly Brady, Obstetrics Floor, Room 203

Goal: To care for a patient with both medical and psychiatric illness, using holistic approaches to manage the patient's stress.

Objectives:

- Describe the physiological manifestations of the fight-or-flight response of the autonomic nervous system when triggered by a stressor.
- Describe some of the common symptoms people experience when they are stressed.
- Identify factors that affect a patient's response to stress.
- Identify the predisposing and precipitating stressors of the patient.
- Evaluate the significance of the patient's stressors.
- Determine the patient's coping styles and resources.
- Identify effective stress reduction techniques and their benefits.
- Evaluate the effectiveness of nursing interventions for individuals' subjective and objective responses to stress.

Exercise 1

Writing Activity

30 minutes

1. Define the fight-or-flight response to stress.

The bodies way of preparing for a situation an individual perceives as a threat to survival — results in increased HR, BP, + CO

2. Define maturational and situational stressors and give an example of each type.

Possibly

1) psychological

???

2) physical

3. In the acute stress (alarm) stage of the general adaptation syndrome (GAS), three principal stress mediators are involved. Match them with their action.

Sympathetic Nervous System Part

Role in the Response to Stress

_C_ Brain cortex and hypothalamus

a. Sends messages to the adrenal cortex

_A_ Hypothalamus

b. Produces corticosteroids to increase muscle endurance and stamina

_B_ Adrenal cortex

c. Signals adrenal glands to release catecholamine adrenalin that increases heart rate, respirations, and blood pressure to enhance strength and speed

4. Factors such as age, sex, culture, life experiences, and lifestyle affect a patient's response to stress. Place an X next to each true statement below.

_X_ Strong social support can act as a buffer against stress.

_X_ Members of many cultures express distress in somatic terms.

_____ Spiritual practices can weaken the immune system.

_X_ Women are more likely than men to assess their own stress as high.

_X_ Proper diet and exercise can help manage stress.

5. List four known benefits of stress-reduction techniques.

- ↓ HR, RR, BP ∴ Improving oxygenation to major organs ∴ ↓ tension

- help manage subjective anxiety + improve appraisals of reality.

- help ↓ stress levels/hormones

6. Cognitive-behavioral techniques are the most effective methods to reduce stress. Match each specific technique with its type of method.

	Specific Technique	**Type of Method**
B	Relaxation exercises	a. Behavioral (body)
A	Breathing exercises	b. Cognitive (mind)
A	Journal writing	
B	Reframing	
B	Meditation	
B	Humor	
B	Biofeedback	
B	Mindfulness	
B	Guided imagery	
A	Assertiveness and problem-solving training	
A	Physical exercise	

Exercise 2

Virtual Hospital Activity

30 minutes

- Sign in to work at Pacific View Regional Hospital on the Obstetrics Floor for Period of Care 3. (*Note:* If you are already in the virtual hospital from a previous exercise, click on **Leave the Floor** and then **Restart the Program** to get to the sign-in window.)
- From the Patient List, select Kelly Brady (Room 203).
- Click on **Go to Nurses' Station**.
- Click on **Chart** and then on **203**.
- Click on **Nursing Admission**.

1. What is the specific aspect of Kelly Brady's history that indicates she has had mental health problems in the past?

   - episode of depression 15 years prior
   - expresses anxiety, "scared to death", about pregnancy.

2. Describe the three recent stressful life events that might contribute to Kelly Brady's depression and anxiety.

   - Pt complicated pregnancy to severe preeclampsia
   - Poor sleeping patterns
   - Mother diagnosed to pancreatic cancer

3. How does Kelly Brady physically express her depression?
   a. Tearfully states she does not want to be alone
   b. Does not show her sadness
   c. Rocks back and forth
   d. Talks with friends

4. Describe stress-reducing techniques you think might be helpful for Kelly Brady.

5. According to the Nursing Admission, what main coping mechanism does Kelly Brady use?

6. How does Kelly Brady feel about her hospitalization?

- Click on **Return to Nurses' Station** and then on **203** at the bottom of your screen.
- Inside the patient's room, click on **Patient Care** and then on **Nurse-Client Interactions**.
- Select and view the video titled **1500: Transfer to Labor and Delivery**. (*Note:* Check the virtual clock to see whether enough time has elapsed. You can use the fast-forward feature to advance the time by 2-minute intervals if the video is not yet available. Then click on **Patient Care** and **Nurse-Client Interactions** to refresh the screen.)

Answer the following questions based on the video you just observed, as well as the information in Kelly Brady's chart and the chapters in your textbook.

7. In terms of Hans Selye's general adaptation syndrome (GAS), what is Kelly Brady's treatment stage?
   a. Acute
   b. Prolonged

8. Given Kelly Brady's stage of treatment, identify the nurse's goal, assessment focus, purpose of interventions, and expected outcomes below.

Nursing goal

Focus of assessment

Purpose of intervention(s)

Expected outcome

9. During the video interaction, what action does the nurse take to indicate she is focusing on the overall goal of stabilization?

10. What does the nurse do to provide Kelly Brady with educational information on the risk factors that are threatening her health and well-being?

11. Discuss the nurse's attempts to manage the environment to provide safety for Kelly Brady.

Anxiety Disorders

Reading Assignments:

Halter: Varcarolis' Foundations of Psychiatric Mental Health Nursing, 7th edition (Chapter 15)

Keltner: Psychiatric Nursing, 7th edition (Chapter 30)

Varcarolis: Essentials of Psychiatric Mental Health Nursing, 2nd edition Revised Reprint (Chapter 11)

Patient: Dorothy Grant, Obstetrics Floor, Room 201

Goal: To care for a pregnant patient who is experiencing anxiety.

Objectives:

- Define anxiety and describe characteristics of generalized anxiety order (GAD).
- Identify stressors leading to a patient's anxiety.
- Define cognitive, behavioral, and physiological responses to anxiety.
- Define defense mechanism.
- Discuss levels of anxiety as they relate to nursing interventions.
- Develop treatment interventions and outcomes for a patient with anxiety.

Exercise 1

Writing Activity

30 minutes

1. Define the characteristics of generalized anxiety disorder (GAD).

2. Anxiety is experienced at different levels. Match each level of anxiety with its characteristics.

Level	Characteristic
_____ Mild	a. The person may demonstrate selective inattention. As the perceptual field narrows, the person focuses on immediate concerns.
_____ Moderate	
_____ Severe	b. Associated with dread and terror, the person exhibits markedly disturbed behavior as the personality becomes disorganized.
_____ Panic	
	c. Associated with tensions of daily life and may produce slight discomfort.
	d. Significant reduction in the perceptual field as the person focuses on specific or scattered details and cannot think of anything else. Learning and problem solving are not possible.

3. Identify at least two physiological responses to anxiety in each of the systems below and on the next page.

System	Physiological Response (Symptoms)
Cardiovascular	
Respiratory	
Gastrointestinal	
Somatic (sensory)	

Genitourinary tract

Somatic (muscular)

4. Describe the automatic coping styles that protect individuals from painful awareness of feelings, conflict, etc., that block personal feelings, conflicts, and memories that can provoke overwhelming anxiety.

5. Specific nursing interventions are key in working with patients to reduce anxiety regardless of the diagnosis. List five of these key nursing interventions.

6. For patients with moderate to severe anxiety, medication may be a necessary intervention. In the table below, list the positive aspects and the cautions associated with the use of antidepressant and anxiolytic medications in patients with anxiety.

Medication Class	Positive Aspects	Cautions
Antidepressants (SSRIs)		
Anxiolytics (Antianxiety agents)		

Exercise 2

Virtual Hospital Activity

30 minutes

- Sign in to work at Pacific View Regional Hospital on the Obstetrics Floor for Period of Care 1. (*Note:* If you are already in the virtual hospital from a previous exercise, click on **Leave the Floor** and then **Restart the Program** to get to the sign-in window.)
- From the Patient List, select Dorothy Grant (Room 201).
- Click on **Chart** and then on **201**.
- Read the **Nursing Admission** record.

1. What are the two stressors listed that contribute to Dorothy Grant's anxiety?

2. One key nursing intervention to reduce anxiety is to encourage patients to discuss their feelings. What does the nurse say to encourage Dorothy Grant to discuss her situation? How does the nurse acknowledge her feelings?

LESSON 5—ANXIETY DISORDERS

3. Dorothy Grant has been using maladaptive coping mechanisms to handle her stressors. For each unhealthy coping mechanism listed in the table below, identify an alternative healthy coping mechanism.

Unhealthy Coping Mechanism	Healthy Coping Mechanism
Hoping the abuse will stop	
Keeping the children quiet	
Blaming herself for causing the abuse (pregnancy)	
Trying not to upset husband	

Copyright © 2017, Elsevier Inc. All rights reserved.

- Click on **Return to Room 201**.
- Click on **MAR** and review Dorothy Grant's medications.
- Check to see whether there are any medications ordered for Dorothy Grant's anxiety.

4. What classification of medications would typically be ordered for a patient with moderate to severe anxiety?
  a. Stimulants
  b. Antidepressants
  c. Antipsychotics
  d. Antianxiety agents
  e. Both b and d

5. Which are important considerations in deciding whether or not to order medications to treat Dorothy Grant's anxiety? Select all that apply.

  _____ She is 30 weeks' pregnant and having possible contractions.

  _____ Her anxiety is initially assessed to be at a moderate level.

  _____ Blunt force trauma to her abdomen may result in preterm birth.

  _____ More time is needed to assess her anxiety level.

6. The best treatment outcomes will demonstrate adaptive ways of coping with stress. From the list below, place an X next to the two statements that best describe desired treatment outcomes based on Dorothy Grant's treatment plan.

  _____ Verbalizes need for assistance, seeks information, and modifies lifestyle as needed

  _____ Identifies and plans coping strategies for stressful situations

  _____ Monitors intensity of anxiety and maintains adequate sleep

  _____ Accepts compliments from others

Depressive Disorders

Reading Assignments:
    Halter: Varcarolis' Foundations of Psychiatric Mental Health Nursing, 7th edition (Chapter 14)
    Keltner: Psychiatric Nursing, 7th edition (Chapter 25)
    Varcarolis: Essentials of Psychiatric Mental Health Nursing, 2nd edition Revised Reprint
           (Chapter 15)

Patient: Kelly Brady, Obstetrics Floor, Room 203

Goal: To care for a patient experiencing a medical health crisis who is also experiencing symptoms of depression.

Objectives:

- Understand prevalence and occurrence of depression.
- Describe common risk factors and precipitating stressors in depression.
- Assess a patient who is experiencing depression.
- Discuss safety as it relates to the treatment of a patient with depression.
- Understand the relationship between depression and pregnancy.
- Describe effective treatments, including pharmacological treatment, for a patient with depression.
- Develop a treatment plan for a patient with depression.
- Plan for relapse prevention for a patient with depression.

Exercise 1

Writing Activity

30 minutes

1. Mood disorders, particularly depression, are common. Which statements regarding depression are correct? Select all that apply.

   _____ Major depressive disorders are twice as common in men as in women.

   _____ Approximately 17% to 20% of Americans will develop a major depression in their lifetime.

   _____ If the first episode of depression occurs in childhood or adolescence, recurrence in adulthood is high.

   _____ The average age for adult onset of depression is the mid- to late 20s.

   _____ Having a positive family history for depression increases one's risk for depression.

2. Depression may result from a complex interaction of causes and common risk factors. Which causes/risk factors can contribute to depression? Select all that apply.

   _____ Negative stressful life events, especially loss and humiliation, or inconsistent parenting

   _____ History of prior depressive episode(s)

   _____ Alcohol abuse/substance abuse

   _____ Brain chemistry abnormalities

   _____ Postpartum period

   _____ Medical illness

   _____ Lack of social support

   _____ Family history of depressive disorders, especially in first-degree relatives

   _____ History of suicidal attempts or a family history of the same

3. Complete the table below and on the next page by listing symptoms associated with persons who have major depression.

Areas to Assess	Symptoms
Affective/emotional	
Behavioral	
Cognitive	
Physical behavior	

Areas to Assess	**Symptoms**
Social	

4. In assessing patients with depression, it is important to think about safety first. Explain the actions the nurse will take to ensure the patient's safety.

5. People with depression have a genuine need to believe that things can get better. Which intervention(s) can help patients with this belief? Select all that apply.

_____　The nurse should initially express hope to the patient.

_____　The nurse should reinforce the fact that depression is a self-limiting disorder and the future will be better.

_____　The nurse should explain to the patient that depression is a chronic disease.

6. There are three phases in treatment and recovery from major depression. Match each phase with its associated intervention approach.

Intervention Approach	**Phase**
_____　Directed at prevention of relapse	a. Acute
_____　Directed at reduction of depressive symptoms and restoration of psychosocial and work function; hospitalization may be required	b. Continuation
_____　Directed at prevention of further episodes of depression	c. Maintenance

7. Successful behavior is a powerful tool to counteract depression. Discuss specific interventions the nurse can make in caring for the depressed patient to effect positive behavioral change. Include three activities the patient can accomplish to make positive behavioral changes.

8. Considering what we know about the clinical course of depression, which measure(s) do you think will help in preventing recurrence? Select all that apply.

_____ Education regarding symptom recognition and seeking help early

_____ Lifetime monitoring and maintenance

_____ Adhering to the treatment regime

_____ Medication, psychotherapy and self-help strategies

9. For treating patients with depression, which class of medication has proven the most effective with the least amount of side effects?
   a. Selective serotonin reuptake inhibitors (SSRIs)
   b. Monoamine oxidase inhibitors (MAOIs)
   c. Tricyclic antidepressant drugs (TCAs)

Exercise 2

Virtual Hospital Activity

30 minutes

- Sign in to work at Pacific View Regional Hospital on the Obstetrics Floor for Period of Care 1. (*Note:* If you are already in the virtual hospital from a previous exercise, click on **Leave the Floor** and then **Restart the Program** to get to the sign-in window.)
- From the Patient List, select Kelly Brady (Room 203).
- Click on **Get Report** and review.
- Click on **Go to Nurses' Station** and then on **203** at the bottom of the screen.
- Now click on **Patient Care** and then on **Physical Assessment**.
- Click on **Head & Neck**.
- Select **Mental Status** (in the green boxes).

1. Based on the mental status assessment, describe two of Kelly Brady's behavioral symptoms.

- Now click on **Chart** and then on **203**.
- Click on **History and Physical** and review.

2. What is the predisposing factor in Kelly Brady's family history related to depression?

3. What is the key fact in Kelly Brady's past medical history related to her depression?

- Click on **Return to Room 203**.
- Click on **Leave the Floor** and then on **Restart the Program**.
- Sign in to work on the Obstetrics Floor for Period of Care 3.
- From the Patient List, select Kelly Brady (Room 203).
- Click on **Go to Nurses' Station**.
- Click on **Chart** and then on **203**.
- Click on the **Consultations** tab and review the Psychiatric Consult.

4. According to information found in the Psychiatric Consult, Kelly Brady has major life events/ precipitating stressors that are contributing to her depression. List several (at least four) major stressors in Kelly Brady's life.

5. To develop a treatment plan to address Kelly Brady's depression, complete the table below and on the next page.

Area	Goal	Interventions
Environment/safety		
Cognitive		

Area	Goal	Interventions
Behavioral		
Social skills		
Education		

6. Discuss how Kelly Brady's current pregnancy difficulties might be related to her depression.

Personality Disorders

Reading Assignments:

Halter: Varcarolis' Foundations of Psychiatric Mental Health Nursing, 7th edition
(Chapters 1 and 24)

Keltner: Psychiatric Nursing, 7th edition (Chapters 9 and 29)

Varcarolis: Essentials of Psychiatric Mental Health Nursing, 2nd edition Revised Reprint
(Chapters 2 and 13)

Patient: Harry George, Medical-Surgical Floor, Room 401

Goal: To care for a patient who is experiencing symptoms of a personality disorder and medical illness.

Objectives:

- Describe the unique traits and characteristics of personality in social and interpersonal functioning.
- Summarize three characteristics shared by people with personality disorders.
- Discuss the common personality traits of individuals with antisocial and borderline personality disorders.
- Describe basic nursing interventions for patients with borderline personality disorders.
- Discuss the nurse-patient relationship when implementing holistic strategies to help the patient's self-management of behaviors.

Exercise 1

Writing Activity

20 minutes

1. Define the term *personality* related to social and interpersonal functioning.

2. Identify the three primary characteristics shared by all personality disorders.

3. Many factors may potentially contribute to personality disorders. Describe these factors in the table below.

Potential Factors	Contributing Characteristics
Genetic factors	
Neurobiological factors	
Psychological influences/environmental factors	

4. The main pathological personality traits of individuals diagnosed with antisocial personality disorder are related to gaining personal power or pleasure without regard for others. What are some specific characteristics of antisocial personality disorder? Select all that apply.

_____ Displays deceitful and manipulative behavior

_____ Conforms to ethical or community standards

_____ Seeks stable relationship with one selected individual

_____ Demonstrates callous attitude/behavior

_____ Demonstrates an absence of remorse or guilt

_____ Engages in impulsive behaviors

_____ Is attentive to own health maintenance

5. The criteria used for defining borderline personality disorder (BPD) include a distorted self-image and a pervasive pattern of unstable interpersonal relationships. What are some additional characteristics of borderline personality disorder? Select all that apply.

_____ Frequent mood changes

_____ Chronic depression

_____ Impulsivity

_____ Suicide-prone behaviors

_____ Separation anxiety

_____ Substance abuse

6. Frequently, individuals diagnosed with borderline personality disorder use a defense mechanism or coping style referred to as splitting. Define *splitting* and discuss how it is used by individuals with BPD.

7. Comorbid and co-occurring disorders are commonly associated with personality disorders. Most people with personality disorders do not think there is anything wrong with them and believe their problems are caused by others. Therefore the disorder is not the initial focus of treatment. What are some of the most common reasons that induce people with personality disorders to seek health care services?

Exercise 2

Virtual Hospital Activity

45 minutes

- Sign in to work at Pacific View Regional Hospital on the Medical-Surgical Floor for Period of Care 1. (*Note:* If you are already in the virtual hospital from a previous exercise, click on **Leave the Floor** and then **Restart the Program** to get to the sign-in window.)
- From the Patient List, select Harry George (Room 401).
- Click on **Go to Nurses' Station**.
- Click on **Chart** and then on **401**.
- Click on **History and Physical** and on **Nursing Admission** and review the information given.

1. Identify the potential stressors that have led to Harry George's current life situation.

2. After reviewing the History and Physical and the Nursing Admission records, list behaviors that may indicate Harry George has co-occurring behaviors that correlate with borderline personality disorder.

3. Harry George comments that he is "a loser" and has been fired from work because of his drinking problem. What other behaviors and characteristics does he display that may indicate he has a borderline personality problem? (*Hint:* Review your text to locate characteristics that relate to a border personality disorder.)

4. Self-care for the nurse is an important element when caring for individuals who have personality disorders. The nurse must be aware of the strong negative emotions these patients may induce. Describe some strategies that nurses can use to monitor their personal stress and establish a therapeutic nurse-patient relationship.

5. Harry George faces an uncertain future as a result of the mismanagement of his diabetes and the long-term complications following his initial leg injury and the development of cellulitis and severe pain. This will result in repeated short-term hospitalizations. His probable inability to stop drinking and impulsive decisions could make him a high safety risk and leave him very vulnerable. Describe the assessments the nurse needs to perform when beginning the nursing process and plan of care for the patient with borderline personality disorder, specifically assessments involving high-risk safety issues.

6. Harry George's repeated short-term hospital stays make setting realistic goals difficult. What education strategies and resources should the nurse and the interdisciplinary team provide in the therapeutic discharge plans for him? (*Hint:* Identify strategies that Harry George needs to do to maintain a healthier lifestyle and manage his physical and emotional health problems.)

LESSON 8

Schizophrenia Spectrum and Other Psychotic Disorders

Reading Assignments:
   Halter: Varcarolis' Foundations of Psychiatric Mental Health Nursing, 7th edition (Chapter 12)
   Keltner: Psychiatric Nursing, 7th edition (Chapter 24)
   Varcarolis: Essentials of Psychiatric Mental Health Nursing, 2nd edition Revised Reprint
             (Chapter 17)

Patient: Jacquline Catanazaro, Medical-Surgical Floor, Room 402

Goal: To care for a patient with chronic schizophrenia who is hospitalized for acute asthma.

Objectives:

- Define schizophrenia and its characteristics.
- Discuss the prevalence of schizophrenia in the population.
- Understand the difference between objective and subjective symptoms of schizophrenia.
- Identify predisposing factors and precipitating stressors of schizophrenia.
- Discuss the focus of treatment for each phase of the illness.
- Identify communication techniques the nurse uses for patients exhibiting the positive symptoms of hallucinations and delusions.
- Describe the importance of education as part of the treatment plan for a patient with schizophrenia.
- Explain the importance of relapse prevention for a patient with schizophrenia.
- Discuss medication as a treatment for patients diagnosed with schizophrenia.

Exercise 1

Writing Activity

45 minutes

1. Provide the definition of schizophrenia and its characteristics.

2. The impact of schizophrenia on the individual and society is enormous. Which statements are true about the prevalence and characteristics of schizophrenia in the population? Select all that apply.

   _____ Men and women are equally represented in the population of individuals with schizophrenia.

   _____ Of people diagnosed with schizophrenia, 100% have the disease for life.

   _____ The most typical onset for schizophrenia is between the ages of 15 or 18 and 25.

   _____ Men have a more severe course; women have more positive symptoms.

   _____ Substance abuse disorders occur in approximately 50% to 70% of individuals with schizophrenia.

   _____ About 10% of those with schizophrenia have nicotine dependence.

   _____ Approximately 1% of Americans will experience schizophrenia in their lifetime.

   _____ Physical health illnesses are more common in people with schizophrenia than in the general population.

3. It is important to understand the positive and negative symptoms of schizophrenia. List the positive and negative symptoms associated with each category below.

Category	Positive Symptoms	Negative Symptoms
Thinking		
Emotion		
Speech		
Behavior		

4. Communication with a patient who has schizophrenia can be challenging. In the table below, list at least three communication techniques that are effective to use with patients experiencing the positive symptoms of hallucinations and delusions.

Positive Symptom	Communication Techniques
Hallucinations	
Delusions	

5. The three phases of treatment for schizophrenia are acute, stabilization, and maintenance. What activity(ies) would accurately reflect the focus during the acute phase of treatment? Select all that apply.

_____ Supervision and structure in a safe treatment setting

_____ Adaptation to deficits

_____ Psychopharmacological treatment in crisis

_____ Medication teaching and side effect management

_____ Complete biopsychosocial assessment

_____ Cognitive and social skill enhancement

_____ Safety assessment and observation

_____ Acute symptom stabilization

6. Discuss the importance of involving the patient and the patient's family in the treatment process.

Exercise 2

Virtual Hospital Activity

45 minutes

- Sign in to work at Pacific View Regional Hospital on the Medical-Surgical Floor for Period of Care 3. (*Note:* If you are already in the virtual hospital from a previous exercise, click on **Leave the Floor** and then **Restart the Program** to get to the sign-in window.)
- From the Patient List, select Jacquline Catanazaro (Room 402).
- Click on **Go to Nurses' Station**.
- Click on **Chart** and then on **402**.
- Click on **Nurse's Notes**.
- Read the admission note for Monday at 1600.

1. What information contained in the nurse's admission note has implications for discharge planning?
    a. Patient has asthma.
    b. Sister is patient's main support.
    c. Patient has no transportation.
    d. Patient has a history of stopping her psychiatric medication.
    e. Both b and d have implications for discharge planning.

- Now read the Nurse's Notes dated Tuesday at 0400.

2. The statement made by Jacquline Catanazaro that people are putting poison into her IV is an example of what type of delusion?
    a. Grandiose
    b. Persecutory
    c. Paranoid
    d. None of the above

- Now read the Nurse's Notes dated Wednesday at 0600.

3. The note describes symptoms of schizophrenia that have a direct relationship to Jacquline Catanazaro's asthma. Explain the relationship.

- Now click on **Consultation**.
- Read the Psychiatric Consult.

4. Identify the positive symptom and two negative symptoms of schizophrenia described in the report.

5. The plan contained within the Psychiatric Consult includes exercise and nutrition. Comment on the relevance of diet and exercise as part of the plan of care for this patient.

- Click on **History and Physical** and review.
- Next, click on **Nursing Admission**.

6. Relapse can be a devastating part of the disease of schizophrenia. For each category below and on the next page, list Jacquline Catanazaro's barriers to compliance that may result in future relapses.

Category	Barriers to Compliance
Health	
Thoughts	
Attitudes	

Category	Barriers to Compliance
Behavior	
Socialization	
Medication	

7. Education will be a critical component of Jacquline Catanazaro's treatment plan. What are her educational needs? Select all that apply.

_____ Healthy living

_____ Medication

_____ Psychoeducation

_____ Illness management

- Click on **Return to Nurses' Station** and then on **402** at the bottom of the screen.
- Click on **Patient Care** and then on **Nurse-Client Interactions**.
- Select and view the video titled **1500: Intervention—Patient Teaching**.
- Now select and view the video titled **1540: Discharge Planning**. (*Note:* Check the virtual clock to see whether enough time has elapsed. You can use the fast-forward feature to advance the time by 2-minute intervals if the video is not yet available. Then click on **Patient Care** and **Nurse-Client Interactions** to refresh the screen.)

8. Discuss the importance of including the patient's sister in the discharge planning and recovery process.

- Click on **MAR** and then on tab **402**.
- Scroll down to locate the antipsychotic medication ordered.
- Click on **Return to Room 402**.
- Click on the **Drug** icon and look up the medication you found in the MAR.

9. Using the Drug Guide, complete the information specified below and on the next page for the antipsychotic medication ordered for Jacquline Catanazaro.

Name of medication

Indication

Mechanism of action

Side effects

Dosage

Nursing considerations

Patient teaching

10. Consider the medication dosage Jacquline Catanazaro is receiving and the usual dosage outlined in the Drug Guide. What might be the rationale for the current dosage the physician is giving to this patient?

Substance Related Disorders

Reading Assignments:
    Halter: Varcarolis' Foundations of Psychiatric Mental Health Nursing, 7th edition (Chapter 22)
    Keltner: Psychiatric Nursing, 7th edition (Chapter 34)
    Varcarolis: Essentials of Psychiatric Mental Health Nursing, 2nd edition Revised Reprint
        (Chapter 19)

Patient: Laura Wilson, Obstetrics Floor, Room 206

Goal: To care for a patient with acute medical needs who also has a diagnosis of polysubstance abuse.

Objectives:

- Discuss the prevalence of drug use in the United States.
- Understand terms associated with addictive disorders.
- Identify precipitating stressors, coping mechanisms, and resources of a patient with polysubstance abuse.
- Identify categories to include in an assessment of a patient with polysubstance abuse.
- Identify key aspects of the treatment plan to include in the education for patients with polysubstance abuse.
- Discuss critical elements of discharge planning for patients who have substance abuse.

Exercise 1

Writing Activity

30 minutes

1. Describe the greatest potential reaction to cocaine, a drug that acts on the dopamine system in the brain and creates pleasurable changes in mental and emotional states.

2. When discussing drug use, terms of abuse are important to understand. Match each term with its corresponding definition.

Term	Definition
_____ Substance abuse	a. Usually moderate to severe physical symptoms that occur when substances are stopped
_____ Substance dependence	
_____ Addiction	b. The coexistence of substance abuse and a psychiatric disorder
_____ Co-occurring disorders	c. Includes withdrawal symptoms and tolerance to substance
_____ Physical dependence	d. Continued use of substances despite related problems
_____ Withdrawal symptoms	e. Primary chronic disease of brain reward, motivation, memory, and related circuitry
_____ Tolerance	f. Result from a biological need that occurs when the body becomes used to having the substance in the system
	g. Physiological reaction to a drug decreases with repeated administrations of the same dose; need more of substance to achieve desired result

3. In addition to taking a history and performing a physical examination, the assessment process for drug use includes laboratory testing. Discuss the importance of drug toxicology testing of patients who present with symptoms of possible substance abuse.

4. Which of the following are possible signs and symptoms of a substance related disorder? Select all that apply.

_____ Drowsiness

_____ Flushed face

_____ Clean and neat appearance

_____ Organized thoughts

_____ Slurred speech

_____ Tremors

_____ Watery or reddened eyes

Exercise 2

Virtual Hospital Activity

15 minutes

- Sign in to work at Pacific View Regional Hospital on the Obstetrics Floor for Period of Care 1. (*Note:* If you are already in the virtual hospital from a previous exercise, click on **Leave the Floor** and then **Restart the Program** to get to the sign-in window.)
- From the Patient List, select Laura Wilson (Room 206).
- Click on **Go to Nurses' Station**.
- Click on **Chart** and then on **206**.
- Click on **Emergency Department** and read the report.

1. What information alerts the nurse that Laura Wilson is abusing drugs? Select all that apply.

_____ Found unconscious

_____ Nausea and diarrhea

_____ HIV-positive status

_____ History of drug abuse

2. The assessment of chemical impairment is complex because the simultaneous use of many substances (polydrug abuse) is becoming more common. Laura Wilson's urine drug toxicology screen came back positive for cocaine and marijuana. Complete the table below and on the next page regarding the characteristics of these two drugs.

Substance	Route	Signs and Symptoms of Use	Withdrawal Signs and Symptoms	Consequences of Use
Cocaine				

Substance	Route	Signs and Symptoms of Use	Withdrawal Signs and Symptoms	Consequences of Use
Marijuana				

- Click on **Nursing Admission** and read the report.

3. In addition to crack cocaine, marijuana, and caffeine, Laura Wilson has also abused two other drugs. What are the drugs identified in the report?

4. No drug can be considered safe when used by a woman during pregnancy. In the table below, list the potential effects on a fetus associated with each substance that Laura Wilson has abused.

Substance	Effect(s) on Fetus
Nicotine	
Marijuana	
Opioids	
Alcohol	

5. The Nursing Admission contains information regarding Laura Wilson's precipitating stressors. Which stressor(s) has she identified? Select all that apply.

_____ Her parents disapprove of her lifestyle.

_____ She is HIV-positive.

_____ This is an unplanned pregnancy.

_____ She needs to quit "crack."

_____ Her boyfriend is out of town.

6. Select the *best* coping resource that is available to Laura Wilson at this time.
   a. Younger sister
   b. Boyfriend
   c. Mother and father
   d. Roommate

7. Describe Laura Wilson's most frequently used coping mechanisms for dealing with her problems.

Exercise 3

Virtual Hospital Activity

30 minutes

- Sign in to work at Pacific View Regional Hospital on the Obstetrics Floor for Period of Care 2. (*Note:* If you are already in the virtual hospital from a previous exercise, click on **Leave the Floor** and then **Restart the Program** to get to the sign-in window.)
- From the Patient List, select Laura Wilson (Room 206).
- Click on **Go to Nurses' Station**.
- Click on **206** at the bottom of the screen.
- Click on **Patient Care** and then on **Nurse-Client Interactions**.
- Select and view the video titled **1115: Teaching—Effects of Drug Use**. (*Note:* Check the virtual clock to see whether enough time has elapsed. You can use the fast-forward feature to advance the time by 2-minute intervals if the video is not yet available. Then click on **Patient Care** and **Nurse-Client Interactions** to refresh the screen.)

1. Which of the statements made by Laura Wilson during the interaction best illustrate her lack of understanding regarding substance abuse?
   a. "The baby will help me stay on track."
   b. "It's not like I'm addicted. I can quit anytime."
   c. "It's not like the baby will be addicted."
   d. "I have quit for a month or two."
   e. All except d.

2. Which statement(s) may indicate Laura Wilson's readiness to abstain from drugs? Select all that apply.

   _____ "It wasn't a hard decision for me. I am looking forward to this baby."

   _____ "I can go for a while without taking drugs."

   _____ "My mom doesn't believe I can do it."

   _____ "I'll do whatever it takes to keep my baby."

3. What do you believe are the barriers to Laura Wilson's abstinence from drugs?

4. Evaluate the nurse's role in educating Laura Wilson on the effects of drug use.

- Click on **MAR**. Verify that you are looking at Laura Wilson's records.
- Locate the medication ordered for pain.
- Click on **Return to Room 206** and then on the **Drug** icon in the lower left corner of the screen. Find and review this medication.

5. Identify the medication ordered for Laura Wilson's pain. In this situation, what are the most important features of this medication in terms of safety?

6. An important aspect of Laura Wilson's treatment plan will be the teaching plan. Match each of the patient's education needs with the interventions that will best help her with that need.

Education Needs	Effective Interventions
_____ HIV-positive status	a. Well-baby clinic and parental support
_____ Caring for the newborn	b. Community AA-based self-help group and individual motivational and cognitive behavioral approaches
_____ Drug abstinence	c. HIV counselor/HIV clinic
_____ Handling family conflict	d. Discuss with hospital social worker/discharge planner
_____ Community resources	e. Family counseling

7. Relapses are common during a person's recovery. Therefore each person must prepare for the possibility of relapse to maintain long-term sobriety. Describe three of the preparation goals/strategies to prevent relapse situations.

8. Relapse should not be viewed as a total failure because it can result in a renewed and refined effort toward change. Identify and discuss the key elements of relapse prevention strategies the nurse can use with Laura Wilson.

9. Community resources will be needed to assist Laura Wilson in her recovery. Select the community resource(s) you think might be helpful to her.
   a. 12-step recovery program
   b. Intensive outpatient program
   c. Relapse prevention group
   d. Individual, group, or family therapy
   e. All of the above

Eating Disorders

Reading Assignments:

Halter: Varcarolis' Foundations of Psychiatric Mental Health Nursing, 7th edition (Chapter 18)

Keltner: Psychiatric Nursing, 7th edition (Chapter 32)

Varcarolis: Essentials of Psychiatric Mental Health Nursing, 2nd edition Revised Reprint (Chapter 14)

Patient: Tiffany Sheldon, Pediatrics Floor, Room 305

Goal: To provide nursing care for a patient with an eating disorder who also has comorbid psychiatric symptoms.

Objectives:

- Discuss the prevalence of eating disorders.
- Identify types of eating disorders and their associated symptoms.
- Identify the predisposing factors related to eating disorders.
- List psychological problems and serious medical complications associated with eating disorders.
- Assess interactions between the nurse and a patient with an eating disorder.
- List the primary goals in the management of a patient with anorexia.
- Develop a treatment plan for a patient with an eating disorder.
- List outcomes for a patient with an eating disorder.

Exercise 1

Writing Activity

20 minutes

1. If a person refuses to maintain a minimally normal weight for height and expresses intense fear of gaining weight, what eating disorder does this person have?

2. The prevalence of eating disorders is on the increase in our culture. In addition, comorbid psychiatric illnesses are high in patients with eating disorders. Place an X next to each true statement regarding eating disorder statistics. Select all that apply.

   _____ Eating disorders are more common among men than among women.

   _____ Most eating disorders begin in the early teens to mid-20s.

   _____ The causes of eating disorders are multifactorial.

   _____ Incidence of obsessive-compulsive personality disorder accounts for 25% of those with anorexia nervosa restricting type.

   _____ The major cause of death in patients diagnosed with eating disorders is suicide.

   _____ Depression and anxiety are common comorbid conditions in people who binge eat.

   _____ A history of childhood trauma and sexual abuse is less common in those with eating disorders than in the general population.

   _____ Fewer than 50% of people with eating disorders seek medical care.

3. Place an X next to the statements below and on the next page that best reflect the most common symptoms of eating disorders. Select all that apply.

   _____ Intense fear of gaining weight; extreme concern about appearance

   _____ Skipping meals occasionally

   _____ Excessive exercising

   _____ Purging through vomiting, laxatives, or diuretics

   _____ Overeating under stress

   _____ Chewing food very slowly

_____ Frequent fasting

_____ Binge or overeating behaviors

_____ Thinking of oneself as fat even though underweight

_____ Comfortable in social settings, especially with the opposite sex

_____ Perfectionist traits

4. Disordered eating can lead to serious medical complications and psychological problems. List some of the medical complications and psychological problems below.

Medical Complications	**Psychological Problems**

5. Many factors can predispose a person to develop an eating disorder. Place an X next to the predisposing factors associated with eating disorders. Select all that apply.

_____ Rigid, meticulous, ritualistic, obsessive-compulsive behaviors

_____ Ambivalent feelings of self-esteem; belief that worth is solely based on appearance

_____ Pervasive sense of ineffectiveness and helplessness; no control over life

_____ Understanding others' feelings and being able to handle one's own intense emotions

_____ Difficulty expressing emotions; rapidly fluctuating moods

_____ Cognitive distortions

_____ History of sexual abuse

6. How do sociocultural factors regarding body size affect the prevalence of eating disorders in adolescent females and women in the United States?

7. Many people who are in treatment for eating disorders have evidence of other psychiatric disorders. Provide the psychiatric comorbidity for each eating disorder listed in the table below.

Eating Disorder	Psychiatric Comorbidity
Anorexia nervosa	
Bulimia nervosa	
Binge eating disorder	

8. Discuss psychological factors, including family issues, that may predispose someone to an eating disorder.

9. What sociocultural biases do you have regarding those who have eating disorders that result in them being severely underweight or overweight?

Exercise 2

Virtual Hospital Activity

15 minutes

- Sign in to work at Pacific View Regional Hospital on the Pediatrics Floor for Period of Care 1. (*Note:* If you are already in the virtual hospital from a previous exercise, click on **Leave the Floor** and then **Restart the Program** to get to the sign-in window.)
- From the Patient List, select Tiffany Sheldon (Room 305).
- Click on **Get Report** and review.
- Click on **Go to Nurses' Station**.
- Click on **305** at the bottom of your screen and read the **Initial Observations**.

  1. Identify behaviors Tiffany Sheldon is exhibiting that may be indicative of comorbid psychiatric disorders.

- Click on **Patient Care** and then on **Physical Assessment**.
- Click on **Head & Neck**.
- Click on **Mental Status** (in the green boxes).

  2. Place an X next to each finding from the mental status assessment that coincides with the shift report and initial observations. Select all that apply.

     _____ Good eye contact

     _____ Listless

     _____ Flat affect

     _____ Energetic

     _____ Avoids eye contact

     _____ Withdrawn

- Click on **Patient Care** and then on **Nurse-Client Interactions**.
- Select and view the video titled **0730: Initial Assessment**. (*Note:* Check the virtual clock to see whether enough time has elapsed. You can use the fast-forward feature to advance the time by 2-minute intervals if the video is not yet available. Then click on **Patient Care** and **Nurse-Client Interactions** to refresh the screen.)

3. Describe your reaction to Tiffany Sheldon's responses to the nurse who is caring for her.

- Click on **Chart** and then on **305**.
- Click on **Physician's Orders** and review the information given.

4. What orders are written that indicate multidisciplinary assessments being implemented for Tiffany Sheldon's care?

- Click on **History and Physical** and review.

5. Describe the three identified medical diagnoses for Tiffany Sheldon.

- Click on **Nursing Admission** and review.

6. List at least two possible psychological (personality traits) and two environmental (family) factors that may be associated with Tiffany Sheldon's eating disorder.

- Click on **Return to Room 305** to exit the chart.

Exercise 3

Virtual Hospital Activity

30 minutes

- Sign in to work at Pacific View Regional Hospital on the Pediatrics Floor for Period of Care 3. (*Note:* If you are already in the virtual hospital from a previous exercise, click on **Leave the Floor** and then **Restart the Program** to get to the sign-in window.)
- From the Patient List, select Tiffany Sheldon (Room 305).
- Click on **Go to Nurses' Station** and then on **305** at the bottom of your screen.
- Click on **Patient Care** and then on **Nurse-Client Interactions**.
- Select and view the video titled **1500: Relapse—Contributing Factors**. (*Note:* Check the virtual clock to see whether enough time has elapsed. You can use the fast-forward feature to advance the time by 2-minute intervals if the video is not yet available. Then click on **Patient Care** and **Nurse-Client Interactions** to refresh the screen.)

1. Tiffany Sheldon's predisposing factors make her especially vulnerable to environmental pressures and stress. Which stressors have contributed to the current relapse of her eating disorder? Select all that apply.

    _____   Parents were divorced 3 years ago

    _____   Family does not understand her problem

    _____   Mom is angry and "disgusted"

    _____   She visited her father in Florida 2 weeks ago

- Click on **Chart** and then on **305**.
- Click on **Mental Health**.
- Read the Psychiatric/Mental Health Assessment.

2. What is Tiffany Sheldon's main maladaptive coping mechanism?

3. For people with anorexia, the issue is not really their weight but rather their control over their own life and fears. Provide an example of this overriding concern that Tiffany Sheldon mentions.

4. In addition to Tiffany Sheldon's nursing diagnosis of Imbalanced Nutrition: Less Than Body Requirements, identify two nursing diagnoses that best describe the psychological components to her eating disorder.

- Click on **Return to Room 305**.
- Click on **Patient Care** and then on **Nurse-Client Interactions**.
- Select and view the video titled **1530: Facilitating Success**. (*Note:* Check the virtual clock to see whether enough time has elapsed. You can use the fast-forward feature to advance the time by 2-minute intervals if the video is not yet available. Then click on **Patient Care** and **Nurse-Client Interactions** to refresh the screen.)

5. One of the most important aspects in assessing patients with an eating disorder is their motivation to change their behavior. What statement does Tiffany Sheldon make that would best define her motivation level? Discuss the impact her motivational level will have in preventing relapse.

- Click on **Chart** and then on **305**.
- Click on **Consultations**.
- Read the Psychiatric Consult.

6. Tiffany Sheldon has two simultaneous plans of care being implemented. One plan involves the eating contract, and the other is the plan devised as a result of the Psychiatric Consult. Complete the table below by identifying interventions for each element of the psychosocial treatment plan.

Psychosocial Treatment Plan	Specific Interventions
Individual therapy	
Family conference/family therapy	
Relationship to eating contract	
Medication	

- Still in the chart, click on **Patient Education**.
- Read the report.

7. Identify the treatment outcomes for Tiffany. Can you think of other important outcomes?

Childhood and Neurodevelopmental Disorders

Reading Assignments:

Halter: Varcarolis' Foundations of Psychiatric Mental Health Nursing, 7th edition (Chapter 11)

Keltner: Psychiatric Nursing, 7th edition (Chapter 34)

Varcarolis: Essentials of Psychiatric Mental Health Nursing, 2nd edition Revised Reprint (Chapter 26)

Patient: Tiffany Sheldon, Pediatrics Floor, Room 305

Goal: To provide mental health nursing care to an adolescent patient.

Objectives:

- Describe the relationship between resilience and stress.
- Understand factors involved in psychiatric disorders of adolescence.
- Understand the developmental tasks of adolescence.
- Identify key areas to include when assessing an adolescent patient.
- Identify signs of mental health when assessing an adolescent patient.
- Explore unhealthy responses to stress by adolescents.
- Describe nursing interventions effective in working with adolescents.
- Explore your own issues when working with adolescent patients.
- Evaluate treatment outcomes for an adolescent patient.
- Explore factors and influences contributing to neurodevelopmental disorders.

Exercise 1

Writing Activity

20 minutes

1. Describe the interaction of factors that cause psychiatric disorders in adolescents.

2. Discuss the concept of resilience and the role it plays in vulnerability to psychiatric disorders in adolescents.

3. Adolescents are concerned about many issues. What are some of the typical issues important to adolescents?

4. Body image, identity, and independence are three issues that can produce a variety of healthy and unhealthy responses as the adolescent attempts to cope with the developmental tasks at hand. Match each issue of adolescence with its characteristics.

Adolescent Issue	Characteristics
_____ Body image	a. Seen as being free of parental control; seeking out adult situations; may become frightened and overwhelmed in the process.
_____ Identity	
_____ Independence	b. Growth and development vary widely; growth is uneven and sudden; compare self to peers.
	c. Childhood dreams end; become negative and contrary; may feel isolated, lonely, and confused.

5. Unhealthy coping responses in adolescence include a variety of behaviors. Discuss the potentially unhealthy responses of adolescents to depression and body image distortion. (*Hint:* Feel free to draw from your own experiences.)

6. Autism spectrum disorders are complex neurobiological and developmental disabilities that are typically diagnosed around the age of 3; however, they may be diagnosed later, when the symptoms limit the child's ability to respond effectively to social demands. The impairments can vary from mild to moderate to severe. Describe at least three related impairments in the following categories.

Social skills

Communication

Behaviors and routines

7. Attention deficit hyperactivity disorder is the most common childhood psychiatric disorder. Most likely, it is a group of conditions rather than a distinct factor in this complex brain disorder. Comorbid behavior disorders are often present, including oppositional defiant disorder or conduct disorder. The symptoms can be inconsistent for some children. What are the criteria for a diagnosis of ADHD to be made?

Exercise 2

Virtual Hospital Activity

30 minutes

- Sign in to work at Pacific View Regional Hospital on the Pediatrics Floor for Period of Care 3. (*Note:* If you are already in the virtual hospital from a previous exercise, click on **Leave the Floor** and then **Restart the Program** to get to the sign-in window.)
- From the Patient List, select Tiffany Sheldon (Room 305).
- Click on **Go to Nurses' Station**.
- Click on **Chart** and then on **305**.
- Click on **History and Physical** and read.
- Click on **Nursing Admission** and read.
- Click on **Consultations** and read the Psychiatric Consult.

1. In working with adolescents, it is important to distinguish between age-expected behavior and unhealthy coping responses. For each issue listed below and on the next page, identify the age-expected behavior. Then, based on your review of the patient's chart, list Tiffany Sheldon's unhealthy coping responses for each issue.

Issue in Adolescence	Age-Expected Behavior	Tiffany's Unhealthy Response
Body image		
Mood		

Issue in Adolescence	Age-Expected Behavior	Tiffany's Unhealthy Response

Activity

2. The specific problems of adolescence that make Tiffany Sheldon a high-risk adolescent are:
   a. substance use and truancy.
   b. severe eating disorder and depressed mood.
   c. suicidal and self-injurious behavior.
   d. problems with conduct and violence.
   e. anxiety and sexual promiscuity.

3. When working with adolescents, it is important for the nurse to understand a few basic principles. Place an X next to the statements that best represent the nurse's understanding of these principles in working with Tiffany Sheldon. Select all that apply.

   _____ Use interventions that promote development of a trusting nurse-patient relationship.

   _____ Provide Tiffany with information about healthy and unhealthy adolescent activities.

   _____ Provide Tiffany written health information only.

   _____ Educate Tiffany on typical teen behaviors.

   _____ Meet with Tiffany only when her parents are present.

   _____ Maintain appropriate treatment boundaries.

   _____ Help Tiffany build healthy coping skills to deal with stress.

   _____ Work to integrate the family's perspective with that of the adolescent.

4. In working with Tiffany Sheldon on the psychological aspects of her unhealthy coping responses, discuss two types of therapy suggested in the Psychiatric Consult and provide a possible rationale for each therapy.

5. Discuss your own feelings about adolescence that might arise in working with a patient such as Tiffany Sheldon.

6. The nurse must objectively evaluate the nursing care that has been provided to Tiffany Sheldon and her family. Which of the following questions would be important to ask in determining whether Tiffany and her family have met the treatment goals outlined in the treatment plan? Select all that apply.

_____ Were Tiffany's and her parents' concerns addressed?

_____ Has Tiffany's problematic behavior decreased and been replaced with more healthy coping responses?

_____ Is Tiffany at 100% of her normal body weight?

_____ Have Tiffany's activities of daily living become more reasonable in intensity?

_____ Do Tiffany and her family have a better understanding of her problems?

_____ Are Tiffany and her parents satisfied with the progress toward treatment goals?

_____ Have Tiffany's interpersonal relationships improved?

Psychological Needs of the Older Adult

Reading Assignments:

Halter: Varcarolis' Foundations of Psychiatric Mental Health Nursing, 7th edition (Chapter 11)
Keltner: Psychiatric Nursing, 7th edition (Chapter 34)
Varcarolis: Essentials of Psychiatric Mental Health Nursing, 2nd edition Revised Reprint
                   (Chapter 26)

Patient: Kathryn Doyle, Skilled Nursing Floor, Room 503

Goal: To understand, assess, and care for the older adult patient.

Objectives:

- Identify factors in later life that contribute to good mental health.
- Identify symptoms of mental illness in the older adult.
- Discuss ageism and how it impacts nursing care of the older adult.
- Understand and use knowledge and specialized skills of the geropsychiatric nurse.
- Acknowledge biases in working with the older adult population.
- Identify components of a comprehensive assessment of an older patient.
- Identify common responses that older adults have in relation to the aging process.
- Plan and coordinate the care for an older adult patient.
- Know effective treatment strategies to use with the older adult patient and family.
- Identify sources of community aftercare support for the older adult patient and family.

Exercise 1

Writing Activity

15 minutes

1. Late-life mental illness is less likely to be accurately diagnosed because of the normal aging processes. What diagnoses for older adult patients would be examples that may have an impact on an accurate mental illness diagnosis?

2. Mental health in late life depends on a number of factors. List some of the factors that can affect the mental health of older adults.

3. Ageism is an important issue that affects how a nurse will care for the older adult patient. Define ageism and discuss its implications for health care delivery.

4. Positive attitudes toward older adult patients and their care must be developed in nursing education programs. Which educational components should be included in a nursing education program? Select all that apply.

_____   Information about the aging process

_____   Discussion about nurses' attitudes toward working with older adults

_____   Exploring the nurse-patient interactions with older adults

_____   Teaching students how to develop sensitivity to the needs of older adults

_____   Developing excellent communication skills with older adults

_____   Discussion of the increased prevalence of older adult patients in hospital beds

_____   Providing respect to older adult patients and appreciating their wisdom and life experience

5. In order to care effectively for older adult patients, the nurse needs to have specialized knowledge and skills. For each of the areas listed below, identify several skills the nurse must have in order to work with older patients.

Area	Specific Knowledge and Skills
Assessment	
Community resources	
Family and/or caregivers	
Medication	
Treatment modalities	
Advocacy	

6. Discuss possible biases you may have in working with older adults.

Exercise 2

Virtual Hospital Activity

45 minutes

- Sign in to work at Pacific View Regional Hospital on the Skilled Nursing Floor for Period of Care 2. (*Note:* If you are already in the virtual hospital from a previous exercise, click on **Leave the Floor** and then **Restart the Program** to get to the sign-in window.)
- From the Patient List, select Kathryn Doyle (Room 503).
- Click **Go to Nurses' Station**.
- Click on **Chart** and then on **503**.
- Click on **Nursing Admission** and read this record.
- Click on **History and Physical** and read.
- Next, click on **Consultations** and read the Psychiatric Clinical Nurse Specialist Consult.

1. The National Institutes of Health recommends a comprehensive older adult assessment that includes assessing the cognitive, behavioral, and emotional status of the older adult. According to the medical record, Kathryn Doyle has depression. Depression is often confused with dementia and is not always recognized. Therefore the nurse needs to be familiar with the symptoms of later-life depression. What symptoms is Kathryn Doyle experiencing that are consistent with later-life depression?

2. In addition to her depression, Kathryn Doyle also seems to be experiencing anxiety. Which of these statements are true regarding anxiety in older adults? Select all that apply.

_____ Comorbid anxiety and depression are common in older adults.

_____ All type of anxiety combined are more prevalent than depression in older adults.

_____ Untreated anxiety can contribute to sleep problems, cognitive impairments, and decreased quality of life.

_____ Anxiety does not affect the family.

_____ Antianxiety medication side effects can result in confusion, oversedation, increased risk for falling, and increased agitation.

_____ Antianxiety medications also decrease depression.

3. Besides interviewing the older adult patient and completing a mental status, there are other key components of the geropsychiatric nursing assessment. For each component listed below and on the next page, include the key elements to be considered. Then list data specific to Kathryn Doyle based on your review of her chart.

Component	Key Elements	Assessment of Kathryn Doyle
Behavioral responses		
Functional abilities		
Physiological responses		

Component	Key Elements	Assessment of Kathryn Doyle
Social support		

- Click on **Return to Nurses' Station** and then on **503** at the bottom of the screen.
- Inside the patient's room, click on **Patient Care** and then on **Nurse-Client Interactions**.
- Select and view the video titled **1150: Assessment—Depression**. (*Note:* Check the virtual clock to see whether enough time has elapsed. You can use the fast-forward feature to advance the time by 2-minute intervals if the video is not yet available. Then click on **Patient Care** and **Nurse-Client Interactions** to refresh the screen.)

4. Depression and sadness are sometimes viewed as a normal part of aging. Kathryn Doyle's response to life events that have occurred over the past 9 months has resulted in a disturbance in her mood. Place an X next to each correct statement as it pertains to Kathryn Doyle's diagnosis of depression. Select all that apply.

_____ The death of her husband has compounded the cumulative losses she has experienced.

_____ She is experiencing prolonged mourning over the loss of her husband.

_____ She demonstrates a loss of interest in her friends and her usual activities.

_____ She is experiencing a loss of independence as a result of her hip fracture.

_____ She has symptoms of fatigue and apathy.

- Click on **MAR**.
- Review Kathryn Doyle's medication list.

5. Does Kathryn Doyle have medication ordered to treat her depression? Discuss the role of medication to treat depression in older adults.

6. Based on the nurse's assessment, Kathryn Doyle has other affective, somatic, stress, and behavioral responses common to older adults. Complete the table below and on the next page outlining Kathryn Doyle's specific issues associated with these common reactions.

Type of Response	Issues Involved with Kathryn Doyle's Response
Situational low self-esteem	

Type of Response	Issues Involved with Kathryn Doyle's Response
Imbalanced nutrition	
Relocation stress syndrome	
Social isolation	

Let's jump ahead in virtual time to observe a later interaction between the nurse and Kathryn Doyle.

- Click on **Return to Room 503**.
- Click on **Leave the Floor** and then on **Restart the Program**.
- Sign in to work on the Skilled Nursing Floor, this time for Period of Care 3.
- From the Patient List, select Kathryn Doyle (Room 503).
- Click on **Go to Nurses' Station**.
- Click on **503** at the bottom of the screen.
- Click on **Patient Care** and then on **Nurse-Client Interactions**.
- Select and view the video titled **1505: Assessment—Elder Abuse**. (*Note:* Check the virtual clock to see whether enough time has elapsed. You can use the fast-forward feature to advance the time by 2-minute intervals if the video is not yet available. Then click on **Patient Care** and **Nurse-Client Interactions** to refresh the screen.)

7. Elder neglect and abuse have become more common in our society because older adults no longer have the status of respect they once had through their extended families. Serving as Kathryn Doyle's advocate, the nurse must be alert for signs of elder neglect, abuse, or exploitation. What are the signs that Kathryn Doyle is being neglected, exploited, or abused?

8. During the family conference, the issue of theft will be addressed. Another concern that will need to be discussed is Kathryn Doyle continuing to live in her son's home after she is discharged from the hospital. For the current living arrangement to work, the environment must include several basic characteristics therapeutic for older adult patients. Place an X next to each critical element you think should be included in Kathryn Doyle's home environment. Select all that apply.

_____ Sense of calm and quiet

_____ Structured routine, usual for her lifestyle

_____ Consistent physical layout

_____ Safe environment

_____ Personal items that provide familiarity and a sense of security

_____ Focus on her strengths and abilities

9. Today, most older adults are cared for in the home. What topics should the nurse include in family education and support sessions that would be critical to Kathryn Doyle's recovery and future?

10. Aftercare for older adult patients is often necessary for a successful treatment outcome. After discharge, what agency support do you think Kathryn Doyle's son will need in the care of his mother in the home?

Cognitive Disorders

Reading Assignments:

Halter: Varcarolis' Foundations of Psychiatric Mental Health Nursing, 7th edition (Chapter 26)

Keltner: Psychiatric Nursing, 7th edition (Chapter 28)

Varcarolis: Essentials of Psychiatric Mental Health Nursing, 2nd edition Revised Reprint (Chapter 18)

Patient: Carlos Reyes, Skilled Nursing Floor, Room 504

Goal: To care for a patient who has neurocognitive impairment and symptoms of cardiovascular disease.

Objectives:

- Compare and contrast characteristics of delirium, dementia, and amnestic disorders.
- Provide examples of severe disturbed behavior associated with dementia.
- Understand underlying principles of nursing interventions for patients with neurocognitive impairment.
- Discuss successful nursing interventions in working with patients with delirium and dementia.
- Identify underlying medical conditions that can produce symptoms of dementia.
- Identify medications used in the treatment of dementia and agitation.
- Provide practical strategies for family involvement in discharge planning and home care.

Exercise 1

Writing Activity

15 minutes

1. What is the common thread in all cognitive disorders in regard to the loss of fundamental cognitive ability?

2. Distinguish between the cognitive disorders of delirium and dementia by matching each characteristic with the disorder to which it applies.

Characteristic	Disorder
_____ Develops slowly over months and years	a. Delirium
_____ Involves multiple cognitive deficits, including impairment in memory without impairment in consciousness	b. Dementia
_____ Short-term memory impaired when assessed during a clear moment	
_____ Always secondary to another condition	
_____ Involves progressive deterioration	
_____ Acute onset; disturbance in consciousness and cognition develops over short period of time; usually hours to days, but can last for months	
_____ Short-term memory lost initially; long-term memory fails slowly	
_____ May be reversible	
_____ Usually irreversible	

3. In addition to the usual dementia symptoms of disorientation, confusion, memory loss, disorganized thinking, and poor judgment, a considerable number of individuals with dementia have secondary behavioral disturbances. Below, match each example to its category of behavior.

Category of Behavior	Example of Behavior
_____ Aggressive psychomotor behavior	a. Incontinence, poor hygiene
_____ Nonaggressive psychomotor behavior	b. Demanding, complaining, screaming
_____ Verbally aggressive behavior	c. Decreased activity, apathy, withdrawal, depression
_____ Passive behavior	d. Hitting, kicking, pushing, scratching, assault
_____ Functionally impaired behavior	e. Restlessness, pacing, wandering
_____ Thought disorder symptoms	f. Hallucinations, delusions

4. Identify at least three nursing interventions to focus on for cognitively impaired patients.

5. Any major imbalance of body functions can disrupt cognitive functioning. Discuss how cardiac disorders and cardiac medications can be potential factors in a diagnosis of delirium.

6. Providing a safe and therapeutic environment for the patient experiencing delirium is very important. Place an X next to each intervention that may be necessary to keep a patient safe. Select all that apply.

_____ Provide reality orientation, frequently as necessary

_____ Communicate often, asking questions in a loud voice

_____ Provide pictures, clock, and calendar as environmental cues

_____ Assist with fluids and meals, toileting, and ADLs

_____ Provide anxiety-relieving medication

_____ Ensure a stimulating, busy environment

_____ Use restraints if necessary, as a last resort

7. What is the major focus of planning the care for a patient with dementia? Identify the nurse's most effective tool in caring for patients with dementia.

8. Which of the following are symptoms that the nurse should look for when caring for a patient with delirium? Select all that apply.

_____ Fluctuating level of consciousness

_____ Slurred speech

_____ Nonsensical thoughts

_____ Day-night sleep reversal

_____ Visual and/or tactile hallucinations

9. In providing care to patients with dementia, priority is given to nursing interventions that maintain the patient's optimum level of functioning. With that in mind, complete the table below and on the next page by listing nursing interventions for each component of care.

Component of Care	Interventions
Communication	
Medications	
Orientation and memory aids	
Toileting	

Component of Care	Interventions
Nutrition	
Wandering	
Agitation	
Family and community	

Exercise 2

Virtual Hospital Activity

15 minutes

- Sign in to work at Pacific View Regional Hospital on the Skilled Nursing Floor for Period of Care 2. (*Note:* If you are already in the virtual hospital from a previous exercise, click on **Leave the Floor** and then **Restart the Program** to get to the sign-in window.)
- From the Patient List, select Carlos Reyes (Room 504).
- Click on **Get Report**.
- Read both shift reports.

  1. As noted in the change-of-shift report, what have been Carlos Reyes' most problematic symptoms?

- Now click on **Go to Nurses' Station**.
- Click on Room **504** at the bottom of the screen.
- Click on **Patient Care** and then on **Physical Assessment**.
- Click on **Head & Neck**.
- Select **Mental Status** (in the green boxes).

  2. From the mental status assessment, what symptoms indicate that Carlos Reyes is having neurocognitive impairments?

3. Place an X next to each behavior Carlos Reyes is exhibiting that is associated with aggression. Select all that apply.

_____ Extreme anxiety

_____ Irritability

_____ Soft-spoken voice

_____ Confusion

_____ Intact memory

_____ Disorientation

- Click on **Go to Nurses' Station** and then on Room **504** at the bottom of the screen.
- Now click on **Patient Care** and then on **Nurse-Client Interactions**.
- Select and view the video titled **1120: The Agitated Patient**. (*Note:* Check the virtual clock to see whether enough time has elapsed. You can use the fast-forward feature to advance the time by 2-minute intervals if the video is not yet available. Then click on **Patient Care** and **Nurse-Client Interactions** to refresh the screen.)

4. Which of the following intervention(s) did the nurse use to respond to Carlos Reyes' agitation? Select all that apply.

_____ Ignored the difficult behavior

_____ Listened to the patient and the patient's daughter

_____ Spoke in a calm, reassuring manner to decrease stress in the environment

_____ Modified the original plan to meet the patient's needs

- Now select and view the video titled **1140: Assessing for Referrals**. (*Note:* Check the virtual clock to see whether enough time has elapsed. You can use the fast-forward feature to advance the time by 2-minute intervals if the video is not yet available. Then click on **Patient Care** and **Nurse-Client Interactions** to refresh the screen.)

5. Assess the son's understanding of Carlos Reyes' illness. What action will the nurse need to take after her brief interaction with the patient's son?

Exercise 3

Virtual Hospital Activity

30 minutes

- Sign in to work at Pacific View Regional Hospital on the Skilled Nursing Floor for Period of Care 3. (*Note:* If you are already in the virtual hospital from a previous exercise, click on **Leave the Floor** and then **Restart the Program** to get to the sign-in window.)
- From the Patient List, select Carlos Reyes (Room 504).
- Click on **Go to Nurses' Station**.
- Click on **Chart** and then on **504**.
- Read the **History and Physical** and review.
- Read the **Nursing Admission** and review.

1. Based on your review of all the pertinent data, what factors may be contributing to Carlos Reyes' confusion? Select all that apply.

    _____   Change in environment

    _____   Recent MI

    _____   History of dementia

    _____   Medication regimen

2. If Carlos Reyes returns to his daughter's home after discharge, discuss the problems that his daughter may have in caring for him.

- Click on **Return to Nurses' Station** and then on **504** at the bottom of the screen.
- Click on **Patient Care** and then on **Nurse-Client Interactions**.
- Select and view the video titled **1500: The Confused Patient**.
- Next, select and view the video titled **1505: Family Teaching—Dementia**. (*Note:* Check the virtual clock to see whether enough time has elapsed. You can use the fast-forward feature to advance the time by 2-minute intervals if the video is not yet available. Then click on **Patient Care** and **Nurse-Client Interactions** to refresh the screen.)

3. Describe the approach the nurse used in dealing with Carlos Reyes' confusion.

4. Interventions that involve family members of patients with dementia are critical to the success of the discharge plan. In the interaction with Carlos Reyes' daughter at 1505, what intervention did the nurse use?

- Click on **MAR** and then on tab **504**.
- Find the medication ordered for anxiety and agitation.
- Click on **Return to Room 504** and then click on the **Drug** icon in the bottom left corner of the screen.
- Locate and review the medication you identified in the MAR.

5. Below and on the next page, provide the information requested for the drug ordered for Carlos Reyes' anxiety and agitation.

Generic name of medication

Class

Mechanism of action

Therapeutic effect

Indication

Dosage

Side effects

Nursing indications

- Click on **Return to Room 504**.
- Click on **Patient Care** and then on **Nurse-Client Interactions**.
- Select and view the video titled **1525: Family Conflict—Discharge Plan**. (*Note:* Check the virtual clock to see whether enough time has elapsed. You can use the fast-forward feature to advance the time by 2-minute intervals if the video is not yet available. Then click on **Patient Care** and **Nurse-Client Interactions** to refresh the screen.)
- Now click on **Chart** and then on **504**.
- Click on **Consultations**.
- Read the Discharge Coordinator Consult.

6. Describe the family conflict associated with Carlos Reyes' care and its importance in planning for discharge. Also describe how the nurse should best approach the family situation.

7. Support for Carlos Reyes' family members will be crucial for their caretaking role. Given the patient's illness and family situation, list the types of community support that will be most beneficial.

8. In successful discharge planning, practical recommendations are necessary for family members who must care for patients with dementia, especially patients who are also agitated and demonstrate aggressive behavior. Considering what you know about Carlos Reyes, provide some practical approaches that you would recommend to his daughter in each area of focus listed below.

Area of Focus	Practical Approaches
Environment	
Communication	
Self-care basics	

Sexual Disorders, Assault, and Violence

Reading Assignments:

Halter: Varcarolis' Foundations of Psychiatric Mental Health Nursing, 7th edition (Chapter 29)

Keltner: Psychiatric Nursing, 7th edition (Chapter 33)

Varcarolis: Essentials of Psychiatric Mental Health Nursing, 2nd edition Revised Reprint (Chapter 22)

Patient: Dorothy Grant, Obstetrics Floor, Room 201

Goal: To care for a patient who is a survivor of family violence.

Objectives:

- Define domestic violence (also called partner abuse).
- Define characteristics common to violent families.
- Describe the stages in the cycle of violence and the role it plays in partner abuse.
- Understand the differences between myths and realities associated with survivors of abuse.
- Discuss the use of empowerment intervention with women who have been abused.
- Describe strengths and coping strategies of someone who is experiencing abuse or violence.
- Discuss nursing assessment and interventions for a patient experiencing family violence.
- Identify central themes in abusive relationships.
- Understand common barriers to battered spouses leaving the abusive relationship.
- Describe critical elements of discharge planning for someone who is being abused.

Exercise 1

Writing Activity

15 minutes

1. Provide a definition of partner abuse or domestic/family violence.

2. Identify the violent behaviors associated with partner abuse (physical, emotional, situational, etc.) What is the underlying desire related to these behaviors?

3. There is a predictable cycle of violence that involves three stages, also described as a process of escalation-deescalation. Match each stage with its characteristics.

Characteristics	**Stage of Violence Cycle**
_____ Perpetrator releases built-up tension by brutal and uncontrollable beatings; severe injuries may result; both victim and perpetrator are in shock.	a. Tension-building stage
_____ Kind and loving behaviors, expressions of remorse, and apologies by the perpetrator; victim believes perpetrator and drops any legal action.	b. Acute battering stage
_____ Minor incidents such as verbal abuse, pushing, and shoving occur; as tension escalates, both try to reduce it; perpetrator may use alcohol or drugs, which makes tension build further.	c. Honeymoon stage

4. There are several myths regarding survivors of abuse. Describe the reality associated with each myth listed below.

Myth	**Reality**
Abused spouses can end the violence by leaving the abuser.	
The victim can learn to stop doing things that provoke the violence.	

Myth	**Reality**
Being pregnant protects a woman from battering.	
Abused women tacitly accept the abuse by trying to conceal it, not reporting it, or failing to seek help.	

5. Strong negative feelings can cloud a nurse's judgment with the necessary assessment and interventions. The attitudes that nurses bring to these situations shape their responses toward survivors of violence. Place an X next to each true statement. Select all that apply.

   _____ Nurses may blame survivors if their behavior leading up to the abuse was questionable.

   _____ Nurses have difficulty understanding why a battered woman will not leave her abuser.

   _____ Nurses may have come from violent environments themselves and identify too closely with the victim.

   _____ Nurses may offer advice and sympathy instead of respect.

   _____ Nurses may have strong feelings of anger toward the perpetrator.

   _____ Nurses have been victimized by violence more often than workers in any other profession.

   _____ Nurses may want to blame the victim for the problems of abuse.

   _____ Nurses who have had clinical experiences with survivors of violence may be less apt to blame than nurses who have not had these clinical experiences.

6. What is your attitude about domestic violence? How was your attitude shaped?

Exercise 2

Virtual Hospital Activity

30 minutes

- Sign in to work at Pacific View Regional Hospital on the Obstetrics Floor for Period of Care 2. (*Note:* If you are already in the virtual hospital from a previous exercise, click on **Leave the Floor** and then **Restart the Program** to get to the sign-in window.)
- From the Patient List, select Dorothy Grant (Room 201).
- Click on **Go to Nurses' Station**.
- Click on **Chart** and then on **201**.
- Click on **Nursing Admission** and review.
- Next, click on **Consultations** and read the Psychiatric Consult and the Social Work Consult.
- Now click on **Mental Health** and read the Psychiatric/Mental Health Assessment, the Depression Inventory, and the Abuse Assessment Screening.

1. Listed below are five types of abuse that can take place within families. Which type(s) of abuse is Dorothy Grant experiencing? Select all that apply.

   _____ Physical

   _____ Sexual

   _____ Emotional

   _____ Neglect

   _____ Economic

2. Dorothy Grant is in one of the special populations that are vulnerable to abuse. Identify this population, as well as the other special populations that are most vulnerable to abuse. What is the most widespread form of family violence?

3. There are general characteristics common to violent families. Below, list the specific characteristics of Dorothy Grant's family that correspond to each of the general characteristics of violent families.

Characteristic of Violent Families	Dorothy Grant's Family
Multigenerational history	
Social isolation	
Use and abuse of power	
Alcohol and drug abuse	

4. What are Dorothy Grant's strengths in dealing with her abusive situation?

5. What are Dorothy Grant's coping strategies in dealing with her abusive relationship?

6. Depression is a common response by women in abusive relationships. According to Dorothy Grant's Depression Scale, what is her level of depression?

Exercise 3

Virtual Hospital Activity

30 minutes

- Sign in to work at Pacific View Regional Hospital on the Obstetrics Floor for Period of Care 2. (*Note:* If you are already in the virtual hospital from a previous exercise, click on **Leave the Floor** and then **Restart the Program** to get to the sign-in window.)
- From the Patient List, select Dorothy Grant (Room 201).
- Click on **Go to Nurses' Station** and then on **201** at the bottom of the screen.
- Click on **Patient Care** and then on **Nurse-Client Interactions**.
- Select and view the video titled **1115: Nurse-Patient Communication**. (*Note:* Check the virtual clock to see whether enough time has elapsed. You can use the fast-forward feature to advance the time by 2-minute intervals if the video is not yet available. Then click on **Patient Care** and **Nurse-Client Interactions** to refresh the screen.)

1. In the video you just observed, the nurse uses therapeutic techniques in an effort to support Dorothy Grant. Below and on the next page, cite specific examples to show how the nurse interacts with Dorothy Grant in the four listed categories.

Category	Nurse's Response
Sharing of knowledge and information with the survivor	
Helping to set priorities	

Category	Nurse's Response
Helping to recognize social influences	
Respecting the survivor's competence and experience	

2. The immediate goal of the nurse in working with Dorothy Grant is to develop trust. In order to develop trust, the nurse must demonstrate nonjudgmental listening and psychological support. How did the nurse accomplish (or *not* accomplish) this in the video? Provide your rationale.

3. Which of the following constraints will make it difficult for Dorothy Grant to leave her husband? Select all that apply.

_____ She is still in love with her husband.

_____ She lacks housing and financial resources.

_____ Her church affiliation supports marriage.

_____ There is a societal stigma attached to abuse and divorce.

_____ Domestic violence reporting is not mandatory in any state.

_____ Her husband is in jail.

4. Dorothy Grant has left her husband twice before and returned. For the battered woman, what do you think is the purpose of this behavior?

5. What is one of the most frightening realities that Dorothy Grant may face in leaving her husband?

6. Several themes expressed by women in abusive relationships have been identified. Knowing the themes Dorothy Grant is expressing will help the nurse in her assessment and interventions. Identify Dorothy Grant's themes below.

Themes of Women Who Have Been in Abusive Relationships	Dorothy Grant's Themes
Lack of relationships outside the home	
Immobility to take action	
Internal feeling of emptiness	
Feeling of being disconnected	

7. Discharge planning will be crucial for Dorothy Grant. Place an X next to each activity that will be necessary for a successful outcome. Select all that apply.

    _____ Create a safety planning checklist.

    _____ Provide her with hotline phone numbers of other survivors of abuse and violence.

    _____ Find a supportive alternate living arrangement for Dorothy Grant and her children.

    _____ Refer her to legal assistance, financial aid, and job training and counseling.

8. Because family violence is a symptom of a family in crisis, what role, if any, do you think family therapy has for Dorothy Grant and her family?

9. Do you believe that Dorothy Grant's current and past responses to the abuse are pathological in nature, or do you think this is the typical way a person would react to physical and emotional trauma? Explain.

Crisis and Disaster

Reading Assignments:

Halter: Varcarolis' Foundations of Psychiatric Mental Health Nursing, 7th edition
(Chapters 16 and 26)

Keltner: Psychiatric Nursing, 7th edition (Chapters 33 and 36)

Varcarolis: Essentials of Psychiatric Mental Health Nursing, 2nd edition Revised Reprint
(Chapters 10, 20, and 23)

Patient: Dorothy Grant, Obstetrics Floor, Room 201

Goal: To provide nursing care for a patient in a health crisis using crisis intervention theory and
techniques.

Objectives:

- Differentiate among the three types of crises and provide examples of each.
- List factors that determine a person's ability to deal effectively with crises.
- Describe the three types of crises.
- Describe the phases in response to a crisis.
- Identify components in a safety assessment.
- Explain the steps involved in crisis intervention.
- List crisis intervention counseling techniques.
- Compare and contrast the differences among primary, secondary, and tertiary intervention.
- Describe counseling strategies associated with each level of nursing care in crisis intervention.
- Recognize disaster occurrences and management of global concerns.

Exercise 1

Writing Activity

45 minutes

1. Everyone can experience a crisis and either struggle to resolve it or make the necessary adjustments to live with it. Provide a definition of a crisis.

2. Below, place an X next to each factor that may limit a person's ability to problem-solve or cope with stressful life events or situations. Select all that apply.

   _____ Concurrent stressful events with which the person is coping

   _____ Quality and quantity of a person's usual coping skills

   _____ Presence of concurrent medical conditions

   _____ Presence of concurrent psychiatric disorders

   _____ Excessive pain or fatigue

   _____ Presence of unresolved losses

3. There are various types of crises. Describe each crisis type listed below and provide an example of each.

Types of Crises	Description and Example
Maturational crisis	
Situational crisis	
Adventitious crisis	

4. To promote safety, what two risk factors should the nurse assess for when caring for a patient in crisis?

5. During a crisis, a person's equilibrium may be adversely affected by a lack of one or more balancing factors. Therefore the nurse must assess the patient for three balancing factors that can help an individual during a crisis. Identify these three balancing factors.

   (1)

   (2)

   (3)

6. Human behaviors that follow a fairly distinct path in response to a crisis event are categorized into four phases of crisis. Below, match each cluster of individual behaviors with its corresponding phase of crisis.

Individual Behaviors	**Phase of Crisis**
_____ Trial and error attempts may fail. Anxiety can escalate to severe and panic status. Automatic relief behaviors of withdrawal and flight may occur.	a. Phase 1
	b. Phase 2
_____ Anxiety stimulates use of problem-solving techniques and defense mechanisms when crisis threatens the self-concept.	c. Phase 3
	d. Phase 4
_____ Anxiety can overwhelm the person and lead to serious personality disorganization, depression, and confusion	
_____ Anxiety increases when defense mechanism response fails. Individual's functioning becomes disorganized.	

7. Crisis intervention entails using short-term counseling to help a patient cope with a crisis. The major focus is on the present problem and includes two initial goals. Identify the purpose of these two goals.

8. List 10 activities the nurse may use when conducting crisis intervention.

(1)

(2)

(3)

(4)

(5)

(6)

(7)

(8)

(9)

(10)

9. The nurse's actions during a crisis remain closely linked to the general nursing process. For each crisis intervention step listed below, identify the corresponding crisis intervention components within the step.

Crisis Intervention Step	Crisis Intervention Components
Assessment	
Possible nursing diagnoses	
Outcomes identification	
Planning and implementation	
Evaluation	

10. There are three levels of nursing care in crisis intervention. Below, match each counseling intervention step with its corresponding level of nursing care.

Counseling Intervention Step

Level of Nursing Care in Crisis Intervention

_____ Provide support for the person who has experienced a severe crisis

a. Primary

b. Secondary

_____ Establish interventions during an acute crisis to prevent prolonged anxiety

c. Tertiary

_____ Evaluate stressful life events the person is experiencing

_____ Ensure the safety of the patient

_____ Facilitate optimal levels of functioning

_____ Teach specific coping skills

_____ Plan environmental changes and make important interpersonal decisions

_____ Assess the problem, support systems, and coping styles

_____ Implement critical incident stress debriefing (CISD)

11. Posttraumatic stress disorder (PTSD) is a global disorder that affects individuals, families, communities, and nations that have experienced or witnessed a highly stressful crisis event. Examples include childhood physical abuse, sexual assault, environmental disasters, combat, accidents and terrorist attacks, or the diagnosis of a life-threatening illness. The common element is the feelings of helplessness or powerlessness. Comorbidities can include depression, anxiety, and substance abuse.

    a. What are two primary symptoms of PTSD?

    b. Identify two nursing interventions that are effective when caring for patients with PTSD.

12. Each large-scale environmental crisis can have a global spiraling impact regardless of where it occurs. Earthquakes, tsunamis, hurricanes, floods, or wildfires can impose significant damage to individuals, communities, and nations. Man-made events (such as technological accidents) and complex events (such as political unrest, wars, and terrorist attacks) are examples of current global disasters. What contributions can the psychiatric and professional nurse provide to disaster preparedness activities related to crisis intervention?

Exercise 2

Virtual Hospital Activity

30 minutes

- Sign in to work at Pacific View Regional Hospital on the Obstetrics Floor for Period of Care 1. (*Note:* If you are already in the virtual hospital from a previous exercise, click on **Leave the Floor** and then **Restart the Program** to get to the sign-in window.)
- From the Patient List, select Dorothy Grant (Room 201).
- Click on **Get Report** and read the shift report.

1. What information in the shift report would alert the nurse that a more thorough psychosocial assessment is needed?

It is important for the nurse to obtain more complete information in caring for Dorothy Grant.

- Click on **Go to Nurses' Station**.
- Click on **Chart** then on **201** for Dorothy Grant's chart.
- Click on **History and Physical** and review.
- Click on **Nursing Admission** and review.

2. In the History and Physical, what information indicates that Dorothy Grant may be in crisis?
   a. Dorothy Grant is 30 weeks' pregnant.
   b. Her husband beat her and kicked her in the abdomen.
   c. Her children are home alone.
   d. Her mother was beaten by her father.
   e. All of the above.

3. The first step in crisis intervention is assessing the patient in five important areas. In the Nursing Admission, what assessment information did the nurse obtain regarding Dorothy Grant's abuse by her husband? Record your findings below.

Element of Crisis Intervention Assessment	Assessment Data Found
Precipitating event	
Perception of the event	
Support system	
Coping resources	
Coping mechanisms	

4. Given Dorothy Grant's perception of the event and her coping mechanisms, what crisis intervention techniques might work best at this time?

5. Provide at least one example of how the nurse could help Dorothy Grant regain her self-worth.